THE COMPLETE BBC DIET

Dr Barry Lynch, who trained in medicine at the universities of St Andrews and Manchester, the Managing Director of the independent television company Prospect Pictures. He is also the author of *Don't Break Your Heart*, *The BBC Diet*, *BBC Healthcheck* and *The New BBC Diet*.

DR BARRY LYNCH

———

THE COMPLETE BBC DIET

PENGUIN BOOKS
BBC BOOKS

The BBC Diet is a healthy way of eating as well as a way of losing
weight but, if you are worried about any aspect of your health, check
with your doctor before starting on this or any other diet

'How long does getting thin take?' Pooh asked anxiously
A. A. Milne

PENGUIN BOOKS
BBC BOOKS

Published by the Penguin Group and BBC Enterprises Ltd
Penguin Books Ltd, 27 Wrights Lane, London W8 5TZ, England
Penguin Books USA Inc., 375 Hudson Street, New York, New York 10014, USA
Penguin Books Australia Ltd, Ringwood, Victoria, Australia
Penguin Books Canada Ltd, 10 Alcorn Avenue, Toronto, Ontario,
Canada M4V 3B2
Penguin Books (NZ) Ltd, 182–190 Wairau Road, Auckland 10, New Zealand

Penguin Books Ltd, Registered Offices: Harmondsworth, Middlesex, England

The BBC Diet first published by BBC Books, a division of BBC Enterprises Ltd 1988
The New BBC Diet first published by BBC Books, a division of BBC Enterprises Ltd 1990
Published together in this revised and updated version as *The Complete BBC Diet*
in Penguin Books 1994
5 7 9 10 8 6 4

Copyright © Barry Lynch, 1988, 1990, 1994
Text illustrations copyright © Penny Saber, 1988, 1990, 1994
All rights reserved

The moral right of the author and illustrator has been asserted

Printed in England by Clays Ltd, St Ives plc

CONTENTS

Acknowledgements

I should like to thank my friends, Suzanne Webber and Chris Weller, for deciding to do this bumper edition of *The BBC Diet*. My thanks go also to the people who worked on the book: Deborah Taylor (Project Editor), Gwyn Lewis (Designer), Kate Gee (Production Controller) and of course the hard workers in the sales team!

My continuing gratitude goes to all at Health Promotion Wales for their help, and in particular to Professor John Catford and Helen Howson. My thanks are also due to Brynda Lewis, a senior lecturer in dietetics, who assessed the calorie counts of all the diet plans.

Above all, I am indebted to my Editor, Susan Martineau, who worked so hard in shaping the book. Her enthusiasm and energy have produced a far better book than I could have achieved on my own.

Introduction

The BBC Diet has sold – in its previous two versions – about two-thirds of a million copies. I'm sure that one of the main reasons for this is that it's a diet that really works. Some of the many success stories of the delighted people who lost weight on *The BBC Diet* are told in chapter 1.

The Complete BBC Diet is a revised and updated version of the previous two books, *The BBC Diet* and *The New BBC Diet*. Here are eight set two-week plans; along with five easy-to-follow flexible plans. A huge choice, which I hope will mean that no one can say that losing weight on *The BBC Diet* is boring! There are also guidelines for a complete DIY version of *The BBC Diet* and exercise programmes for shaping your body and really getting it to look good.

The BBC Diet is both a healthy way of eating and a surefire way to lose weight. It's been proved that the very best way to lose weight is also the healthiest: by eating less fat and less sugar and by eating more fibre – and starting to take some exercise.

We make no claims that *The BBC Diet* is a 'miracle' one. The truth of the matter is (and few diet books dare say this) that there is no miracle diet. What we do claim, though – and have proved – is that it works.

Being overweight can be explained in one sentence. If you take in more energy (calories) in your food than your body needs for your particular lifestyle, then your body will lay down that surplus energy as fat. The *only* way to lose weight is to take in less energy or to expend more. Please, please don't let anyone tell you differently. So many people want to believe in a magic 'something' which will help them lose weight but it doesn't exist.

No one can claim we know all there is to know about nutrition, obesity and healthy eating as there are still gaps in our knowledge. But what can now be confidently asserted is that the healthiest diet – the one which most reduces the risk of a wide range of diseases – is also the safest and most effective one to return you to your ideal weight and keep you there. This is good news – after all, everyone wants to be slim and healthy, not thin and ill.

Any books or articles written about dieting tend to take one of two extreme views:

* The 'too much dieting can make you fat' camp which states that all diets are basically a con (but go on to explain that a *healthy* pattern of eating can make you slim).

* The 'lose 2 stone in a fortnight' camp which states that *this* is the diet you've been longing for: in a few short weeks you will have lost weight, found fame, fortune and happiness, and will never have to think about food again!

The BBC Diet tries to steer a middle course between these two extremes. It's not true that all diets are a con, but it is true that to lose weight permanently you have to understand something about your pattern of eating and shape it, long term, into a more healthy – and therefore more slimming – one. It's not true you can lose 2 stone, or anywhere near it, of *fat* in a fortnight (that's a scientific impossibility!) though it is true that a good diet will help you lose a morale-boosting amount of *weight* in those first couple of weeks. (See pp. 45–6 for the difference between losing *fat* and losing *weight*.) What you need to know though, is that it's natural – indeed inevitable – that that rate of weight loss will slow down, but you can continue to lose weight steadily and *maintain* your weight loss. *The BBC Diet* tells you how.

To lose weight successfully – and to keep it off – you need to know why you got fat in the first place.

You need to *know* about food – which foods are packed with calories, which are not – so that you're armed with the knowledge that enables you to fight the flab. *The BBC Diet* teaches you some simple, general principles which, once you know them, give you the power to change your life forever. Then you won't be tied to calorie tables and you won't be at the mercy of fad diets, but you will be in charge of what you eat, and in charge of your own body.

If you're fat, there's no need to be fatalistic about it. Getting slim is within your reach: it's within everyone's reach. It's harder for some people than it is for others but it is possible for all. As I said earlier, I don't promise miracles, but I do promise you this: if you follow the advice in this book, you needn't be hungry, you can still enjoy food and you *will* succeed in getting slim.

Now there's an offer you can't refuse!

1 They Did It – So Can You!

The BBC Diet really, really does work – as has been shown by the very many letters of delight and appreciation we've received since the first *BBC Diet* book was published.

We did know that it worked, though, as we'd already tested it. With the help of our friends from Heartbeat Wales, the heart disease prevention programme of Health Promotion Wales, we got a hundred-strong studio audience to test the diet while *The BBC Diet Programme* television series was being recorded. Over four weeks our highly mixed audience shed a total of 850 lb – that's an average of over half a stone each. We followed up some of our 'guinea pigs' in more detail and there were spectacular weight losses of 2, 3 and even 4 stone.

Much to many people's surprise, even the programme's co-presenter, the wonderful singer Barbara Dickson, has to watch her weight.

When I was invited to co-present The BBC Diet Programme *I thought I knew everything about diets! Like most women, I had tried every fad and trend to achieve the body beautiful. The BBC Diet taught me what I knew all along in my heart, that diet and fitness are all about sensible eating. Fat and sugar make you fat, and that's, I suppose, the rule. I still like fat, but now I'm careful with the family consumption of it with low-fat spreads, semi-skimmed milk etc. Those are for us these days, but mayonnaise in*

*moderation is also allowed – a little of what you fancy! I'm
delighted to see a vegetarian section of the diet in this new
book with so many of us now not eating meat. Bon appétit!*

Roy Noble, Barbara's co-presenter of the series, lost 2 stone
on *The BBC Diet*. He followed the diet with the studio
audience.

*My jowls have disappeared and I've discovered the joys of
the double-breasted suit. I'm now a fan of boiled potatoes
and rarely miss chips – though I do have the odd chip now
and again for a 'taster'!*

*My wife is delighted with my new image, but I now
wonder if my head looks too big for my diminished body. My
hair goes further though!*

I CAN'T BELIEVE IT, I'M A TOTALLY DIFFERENT PERSON

Gillian Jenkins from Penarth in South Glamorgan was one
of our television audience slimmers. It was a huge delight for
me to see how much weight she lost – but, of course, a much
bigger delight for her!

*I'm 29 and I'd been overweight since I was seven. When I
started The BBC Diet I was 15 stone 4 lb and I really felt
miserable. I felt so unfit and I had no confidence in myself.
If my husband wanted to go out, it would take me two hours
to come round to the idea and, of course, I never had
anything to wear.*

*I'd tried so many diets. I bought every diet book going, but
they were all either too faddy, too expensive or I just couldn't
be bothered with them. I tried them for a couple of days but
gave up – I'm not at all strong-willed. I'd been to one
slimming club, lost 2½ stone, but then put it all back on
when I stopped. I went to another club, lost 2 stone, stopped
and put it all back on.*

The secret of my success with The BBC Diet *is that it's so easy – it's unbelievably simple. When I started it and went shopping I couldn't believe what I could eat, it was incredible. So I didn't need any willpower.*

I've now lost 4½ stone and it's stayed off and I'll be happy if I lose another few pounds. The great thing is, it's all shifted from my hips and bottom. From my waist I've lost only 4" going from a 32" to a 28" but from my hips I've lost an incredible 12" going from 52" to 40". It's a joy now to buy clothes off the peg and a couple of months ago I bought my first ever pair of jeans – at the age of 29! I thought I'd won the pools.

I can't believe it really – I'm a totally different person. I feel fabulous, I feel so well. I've got bags of confidence. I've now got a job – I never had the confidence to work before. My outlook on life has changed totally. I now run twice a week and swim with the children and really enjoy it. Before, the only exercise I did was walking upstairs. I feel now that life is for living and if I want to do something, I'll go for it. I found people treated me horribly when I was fat – you feel disregarded, pushed in the background. It's amazing that people now do treat me differently.

My husband is absolutely thrilled. I'd been on so many other diets that when I began this he thought 'here we go again'. But once I'd lost over 2 stone he knew it was different. Sometimes I see him looking at me and say 'What are you looking at?' and he says 'I'm just looking to see if it's still you!' My mother, who's a nurse, is so pleased too. Her friends say I now look like her, which I never did before.

I know the weight's going to stay off because I've changed my whole attitude to food. I know I'm eating more healthily all the time now. I'd say to anyone 'just try The BBC Diet. *Don't think about it – just do it.'*

Apart from the success of our television 'guinea pigs', here's a selection of some of the many encouraging letters we received.

IT WAS SO EASY

Colin and Kathleen Mileham from Great Yarmouth were one of many married couples who wrote to tell of their joint success on *The BBC Diet*. In Colin and Kathleen's case, their joint weight loss was a staggering 7 stone 7 lb! Kathleen, who's 51, went from 14 stone 2 lb to 10 stone 9 lb. She's 5' 4". The 'Middle Way' they mention is also equivalent to the Easy Way, Vegetarian, Gourmet or No-bother Plans in this book.

> *We followed the 'Middle Way' plan, and it was so easy. I felt we were eating so much of the food we would normally eat anyway. I hardly ever felt hungry and I even did give myself the odd treat, like a scone. All our friends noticed how much weight we've lost and there were comments like 'my goodness, you are getting slim'. I've had to have all my clothes taken in, of course. I've gone from a size 20 to a size 14 now for skirts and trousers and a bust size 16. I feel so much fitter now. Before, I had difficulty walking uphill but now I swim regularly and I walk our two dogs twice a day. I really think The BBC Diet is great and I'd recommend it to anybody. As for my husband, he's feeling very pleased with himself.*

Colin is 54 and 6 foot tall. He's gone down from 16 stone 11 lb to 12 stone 11 lb – a loss of 4 stone.

> *The doctor had been on at me for years and years to lose weight because of my arthritis and so I decided to start on The BBC Diet with Kathleen - and it was so easy. I certainly feel different in myself and I can move better. One of my daughters and my son said how much better I looked*

for it - my other daughter wondered halfway through if I'd already lost enough!

My wife and I put a chart of our weight on the wardrobe door - and I'm afraid, despite what you said in your book, we weighed ourselves twice a day! It was great doing it together. I lost weight steadily every couple of days whereas my wife did find she went through a plateau of a week or so of not losing weight, and then suddenly she would lose some more.

So, The BBC Diet certainly worked for us with no problems at all. The great thing about it was you're not forced to eat loads of salads which I would have found boring - I liked the meals I had. It's changed the way we shop - we have wholemeal bread which I now prefer to white and we also have much more fresh fruit.

YOU'VE GOT ANKLES AGAIN!

That was the delighted exclamation of Maureen Handley's husband. Maureen, who's 62, has lost nearly 3 stone on *The BBC Diet.* She's 5′ 3″ and has gone down from 16 stone 2 lb to 13 stone 3 lb and is really feeling pleased. She wrote to me from her home in New Malden to tell her story.

I started putting on a lot of weight in my 40s. I was size 24 and I went to buy a new dress and I realised I needed a size 26 and I thought 'Oh no, you don't!' I then saw The BBC Diet television programme and decided to follow it.

I found it easy and had no problems. I couldn't have done it if I'd been told to eat just salads — I'd have felt awash with them. Making my mind up that I was going to succeed was a big help. I was surprised but I really wasn't hungry. I used to like sweets and chocolate but I'm amazed at how I haven't missed sweet things. I found following the guidelines of less fat and sugar and more fibre was easy, even while having to cook for someone else.

Now I don't have to hunt around for outsize dresses and that makes me really pleased with myself – and seeing the weight drop off my hips, thighs and ankles was great, and was appreciated by my husband too! I've noticed my knees, which used to be painful, now feel great and I've realised that I'm walking faster than before. I can even run for a bus now! I feel healthier. I'd started getting dizzy when I stood up but all that's gone now. And the comments I got! 'Your dresses look big!' was the best one.

I think The BBC Diet is so good, the guidelines were just right for me – I didn't feel I was being watched. I keep telling people about it and I'd recommend it to anyone.

I'M DELIGHTED

So said 31-year-old Melanie Reidy from Cardiff.

I've lost 1 stone and 4 lb. I'm 5′4″ and I've gone down from 12 stone to 10 stone 10 lb – I lost 12 lb in the first month. I'm very pleased with what I've done so far and now I'm determined to lose another 10 lb to get to my target of 10 stone. I've totally changed my eating habits and I'm delighted. My husband followed the diet with me although he didn't really need to lose much! He's 5′9″ and has gone down from 13 stone 1 lb to 12 stone 7 lb.

I've been so enthusiastic I've even started a slimming club in my road. I extol the virtues of The BBC Diet's guidelines – less fat, less sugar and more fibre – which is, of course, just sensible eating really. My neighbour has now lost 1 stone 2 lb and so that's another incentive for me to get down to my target. The problem has been that so many people said to me how well I've done, that I was in danger of getting a bit complacent!

I'VE NEVER TRIED SUCH AN EASY DIET

Hilary Wade wrote to me from Lincolnshire. She works from home as a music agent booking string quartets and orchestras around the world. She followed The Short, Sharp Shock which is equivalent to the Quickfire Plan.

I moved to Lincolnshire from London and promptly put on 2 stone. I found if you went to someone's home you'd be offered cakes and an immense amount of food and it was difficult to refuse. I'm 5'6" and I'd gone up to 12 stone. My daughter is a nurse in a coronary care unit and she'd gone on at me to lose some weight. I'd tried slimming clubs and other diets, but nothing worked until I tried The BBC Diet.

I'd gone on holiday to Rye and went into a bookshop. There was a big pile of BBC Diet books with a handwritten notice above: 'Our customers love this book'. I thought to myself 'Well, I'd better have a go at this'.

I think The BBC Diet is so sensible – it's down to earth and there's no nonsense. It doesn't ask impossible things of you and it's jolly easy to follow – in fact I've never tried such an easy diet. The menus are so good and, although I've got a busy job, the meals are easy to cook. On other diets I'd felt hungry, but not on this. I followed The Short, Sharp Shock and I lost 6 lb in the first week. I then lost 1 stone 7 lb in less than 4 months. I felt I was eating quite a lot and I certainly didn't feel deprived.

I've lost at least 3" off my waist and of course my daughter is very pleased. I'd lost weight before with slimming clubs but had quickly put it on again. That certainly hasn't happened with The BBC Diet. It is really lovely still to cook from the book.

MY WIFE SAYS 'I'VE GOT A NEW MAN!'

'No one likes to be fat and the way you talked about losing weight in your book made me realise that I needn't continue to be fat.' That's what Neil Sansom, a 42-year-old production director for a printing firm, told me.

I was 16½ stone and as I'm 6′ 2″ I carried my weight reasonably well. But secretly I really felt unhappy about it – I felt slow and lethargic and I was embarrassed to go swimming. I'd tried to diet before and my weight would go down and then I'd put it all back on again.

I read The BBC Diet *book and it was so sensible – it just felt right. I started on it and in the first week I lost ½ stone. I couldn't believe it. Since then I've lost between 1 and 5 lb a week for the last 3 months. I've now lost 3½ stone so I'm down to 13 stone.*

I couldn't have followed a rigid diet but The BBC Diet *is so flexible. It was so easy and I never felt hungry – in fact I was eating more potatoes than I ever had in my life! I'd been a foodaholic all my life but eating all the wrong foods, and suddenly I now wasn't. It all made such sense to me – cut down the fat and sugar and increase the exercise. It's commonsense: you must lose weight, but you put it in such a way that I really could believe it.*

I used to get breathless walking but now I cycle 3 miles three or four times a week. For the first time ever, I'm buying my clothes off the peg. My friends have been quite amazed and one or two said 'You'll never keep it off'. But I have done. Unless you've been fat you can't appreciate it, but I never ever want to get fat again. My wife is so chuffed she says she's got a new man. I feel a new man. I looked at myself in a mirror the other day and suddenly realised I didn't have that huge stomach hanging in front of me. We've just come back from a holiday in France and I've just seen the photos. I hardly recognise myself. For years I fought shy of cameras and suddenly I thought 'This doesn't look like me – thank goodness!'

I'VE PLUGGED IT LIKE MAD

Those were the kind words of Yvonne White who wrote to me from Bushey, Hertfordshire.

I think The BBC Diet *is fantastic. I must say, I'm highly delighted with the results of following it. The BBC Diet suited me - I would never have followed a calorie-counting diet or regular meetings with other dieters.*

I watched the television programme and started dieting in the middle of January 1989 when I was a disgusting 11 stone 3 lb – I'm 5' 3" – and I was most unhappy. I was full of aches and pains, 20 minutes walking around Watford shopping was a misery, climbing the stairs to the car park was out, I always took the lift whenever possible and the thought of a long walk was a nightmare. I got the book, The BBC Diet *and read it, several times in fact. At first I thought 'I'll never do it', but I wrote down in an exercise book the menus I was going to use.*

But then I realised I was losing a steady 2 lb a week and this spurred me on as I could see that it really did work and, more to the point, without any discomfort or longings for things I had given up.

I tried to combine a little bit more exercise with the diet, for example, not just walking up to the post office for the paper, but going 'the pretty way' - right round the block - at a good brisk pace. It was surprising how soon I could walk that distance without puffing.

I'm now 9 stone 5 lb - I've lost 2 stone 12 lb! To be able to eat baked beans for lunch or a low-fat burger is incredible. In some cases I find that I'm eating more than I did before, but without that over-indulged feeling.

I've had so many congratulations and even some remarks

of 'Don't lose any more!' And I can honestly say that it hasn't been a struggle or in the least painful. In fact, I really enjoyed doing it if the truth were known! Lots of aches and pains have gone and I feel so much better - walking is a pleasure now and not a chore. So it's worked wonders for me. I've plugged it like mad. I must have sold half a dozen books. It's first class and I'd recommend it to anyone.

I USED TO YO-YO BETWEEN LOSING WEIGHT AND PUTTING IT BACK ON AGAIN

Joanna Wimbush of Berkhamsted lost 1 stone 8 lb on *The BBC Diet.*

I'd been overweight since the age of 13 and for years I'd followed one diet or another, always losing weight but always putting it back on until . . ., as the storybooks say, I was lucky enough to read about The BBC Diet in Radio Times. I bought the book and followed it – with excellent results.

I lost a stone in a month as well as inches all round and continued to lose weight the next month although easing myself off the diet – and I've not put it back on. This was the first diet I'd followed where friends said 'You're looking great'. Before when I'd lost weight, they would say 'You're not looking well'!

Now I weigh 10 stone 10 lb and I've never been down to that since I was 13. I feel so well. Before, I was lethargic and didn't want to do anything. My friends say I look better than I have for years. I've lost 4" from my waist and 4" from my thighs. I was struggling to get into an 18 dress size – I was really size 20 – and now I'm a comfortable 16. It's lovely to go into those posh ladies' shops where the assistants used to say to me snootily, 'Oh no, nothing over 16'.

And your diet is so easy! It's the easiest thing in the world. I can't tell you how many people I've recommended it to.

The local bookshop must wonder what's going on. I was working in Strasbourg recently and I gave my copy to someone there. She put her French husband on it! Well done: many thanks.

CONGRATULATIONS ON YOUR WONDERFUL EFFORT TO GET THE NATION LOOKING FIT!

That was the opening line of a letter from Gerald and Joan Barber who live in my home town of Salford in Greater Manchester. They were another married couple who followed the diet together. Gerald Barber lost 7 lb in his first week on *The BBC Diet.*

It's the finest diet anyone could follow. I've now lost a total of 1½ stone and I feel 100 per cent fitter – I do honestly. I suffer from arthritis and that's so improved, I can now walk anywhere. Everyone's remarked how much slimmer and younger we're both looking. No wonder – my pot belly's gone and my wife has lost inches all round including 4" from her hips.

Joan Barber finds she can now walk and go shopping without getting breathless.

I've lost 1 stone 3 lb and my big spare tyre has gone. I feel a lot better. I used to have such a sweet tooth – biscuits, chocolates, anything – but I've stopped all that. But I didn't feel at all deprived. I was never hungry and we felt as if we were eating good meals. It's such a good diet – I'd recommend anyone to follow it. You won't feel as if you're having to go without!

IT'S THE BEST DIET I'VE EVER USED

So wrote Jan Seaman from Huntingdon in Cambridgeshire.

It's very sensible and it's so down to earth and easy to follow.

My husband enjoyed the recipes and partly followed the diet with me – he lost 1 stone. I've lost 1 stone as well and I've gone from a 16 dress size to a 14 and sometimes a 12. Once or twice I felt hungry on the diet, but I'm greedy and I love my food. My husband never felt hungry at all!

What impressed me was that I didn't have to race around to find difficult foods – I'm very busy in the week and the foods were easy to shop for and easy to cook. It's an interesting diet and the recipes are so economical.

I was so fed up before I started the diet. I couldn't get into half my clothes. I feel so much better, definitely.

I FEEL IN CONTROL OF MY LIFE AND MY BODY

Patricia Manchee from Glossop in Derbyshire teaches embroidery and dressmaking.

And before I went on The BBC Diet, I had to make all my clothes as it wasn't worth going into a clothes shop. I'm 5′4″ and I was 14½ stone. I used to be a great eater of Mars bars and chocolate for comfort.

I'd tried other diets, in fact I was an inveterate dieter. But I'd lose weight, put it on again and then give up. It was different this time. I found this was a diet that really works. I've lost 3½ stone with The BBC Diet – and I've kept it off. The BBC Diet helps you to think what you're doing and it teaches you a new way of eating.

People are amazed at my new looks and remarks of 'Good heavens' were common! I feel so much better. It's improved my self-confidence – I feel in control of my life and my body.

I enjoy walking now. I feel younger and fitter.

I now dress differently. I used to try to look like a semi-smart matron but now I've dared to wear things like printed trousers and even trainers! I'm afraid I now do tend to look into other people's shopping trolleys at the supermarket and think 'How funny to be eating all that!' And those were the very things I used to eat myself which made and kept me fat!

Patricia's target is to lose another stone – and she's certainly on course.

2 How Fat is Fat and Does It Matter?

'TELL ME WHAT YOU EAT AND I WILL TELL
YOU WHAT YOU ARE.'

BRILLAT-SAVARIN

How many people do you know who are trying to lose weight at the moment? Or is an easier question, how many people do you know who are *not* trying to lose weight at the moment? It's been reported by the advertising industry that, at any one time, 65 per cent of British women and 30 per cent of British men are trying to lose weight. A third of the population are also regular users of one or more slimming products. It seems that it's the norm in this country to be overweight. There is, as doctors often say when confronted with something they don't understand, a lot of it about!

This chapter tells you how to recognise if you're 'officially' overweight and what those 'what you should weigh' charts really mean. It also details the medical risks associated with being fat and considers our attitudes to obesity and body shape.

If you know you're overweight, know you want to lose weight and don't want to know about medical risks, you can jump to the next chapter which tells you why nature or fate has picked you out to be fat and not your thin friends.

26

Most people know only too well whether or not they are overweight – and know what weight they would like to be and feel comfortable at. But in case you are wondering – or perhaps hoping! – here are two quick ways of determining *if* you are overweight.

'Pinch an inch'

Whilst standing, loosely get hold of the skin at the side of your body at waist (navel) level. Use your forefinger and thumb and just get hold of the skin – not a great wodge of underlying flesh.

Well? If this pinchful is an inch or more, you're overweight and could do with losing some.

The mirror test

Take all your clothes off and stand in front of a full-length mirror. Take a good look at yourself. Perhaps that's enough and you don't need to go any further, but the idea here is to jump up and down on the spot gently, taking a hard look at yourself as you do.

Are you lithe and taut or are there definite wobbles? Wobbles – and particularly bits of you taking on a life of their own and perhaps moving at different speeds! – mean you definitely need to shed a few pounds.

THE SCALE OF THE PROBLEM

On the basis of the statistics above, at least two-thirds of women and one third of men 'know' they're overweight but decide to do nothing about it. More objective evidence confirms the massive scale of the problem: about half of the middle-aged people in this country may be classified as being above their ideal weight.

HOW OVERWEIGHT ARE YOU?

Take a look at the height/weight charts on p. 30 and see which band you land in and whether you're on the good or bad side of that band or in the middle. These charts offer a 'desirable weight' band which, as you can see, is quite broad. The charts are based on life assurance tables and the 'desirable' band is associated with the lowest death rates: they give only an approximation of how fat or thin you are as, of course, body fat and weight are not exactly the same thing. It is possible for some people to be heavy in weight, but not very fat because of large, well-developed musculature. Most of us, though, don't need to worry about such things: on the whole, if we are overweight, we are fat. But the tables are on the generous side: you can be 1 or 2 stone overweight and still be quite healthy (though after that, your health may certainly start to suffer) but, of course, you may not be happy with yourself at this weight. So these tables are really only a very rough guide. The desirable weight for you is the one you feel most happy at. For your health's sake, though, it shouldn't be much less than a few pounds below the bottom of the desirable band. But probably most women, and even some men, are certainly going to feel happier if they are at the lower edge of 'desirable'.

BODY SHAPE

There is of course an intimate connection, though not a completely direct relationship, between our weight and the shape of our body.

When men lay down surplus fat, they tend to become 'apple-shaped', put on fat around their middle and develop a paunch. When women lay down fat, they tend to become 'pear-shaped'. Under the influence of the female sex hormones, fat tends to get laid in the hips, thighs and buttocks. Many myths have grown up about this type of fat: for example, it's completely different from 'ordinary' fat (sometimes it's called cellulite); it can be shifted specifically by special diets; it's much harder to get rid of than 'ordinary' fat; it can be got rid of by massage or by rubbing special creams into the skin; it's impossible to shift that last pound or two of it.

These *are* all myths. Under the microscope, this fat is exactly the same as any other fat and it is laid down and can be shifted in exactly the same way as any other fat. Being told to use massage or creams or specific diets is hocus pocus!

Any diet which works – that is, any diet which effectively cuts calories – will cause the fat in the body stores to disappear, wherever it is. And in men it tends to be in the paunch and in women on the thighs and hips.

We all come in different shapes and some people may have to accept, even if they have lost the weight they wanted to, that they do not achieve the absolutely perfect shape they want to be. After all, not everyone is happy with the shape of their nose! And so it is with hips, or any other bits of the body.

However, you can *improve* your shape by losing weight, and particularly by exercising to start toning up your muscles. Ordinary exercises like walking and swimming help to tone up all the muscles in your legs and buttocks, but in chapter 21 there are some suggestions for specific exercises which will help to tone up your tummy, your thighs or your hips.

HEIGHT-WEIGHT CHART

Find where you are on the chart by taking a line from the left-hand or right-hand side which gives your height. Follow this until it meets your weight line coming from the base or top of the chart on the next page.

MEN

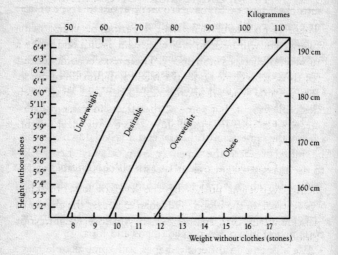

WOMEN

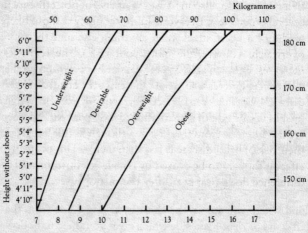

THE MEDICAL RISKS OF OBESITY

There is no doubt that, over a period of years, being overweight will have an effect on your health and make a number of diseases more likely. These risks become serious for those who come under the medical definition of obese, that is those who are more than 20 per cent above their desirable weight, but some of the effects increase progressively when you are just slightly above your ideal weight.

Overweight and raised blood cholesterol

Being overweight pushes up the level of fats, including cholesterol, in the blood. This then increases the chance of a heart attack or a stroke. When you lose weight, your blood cholesterol level falls.

Overweight and heart disease

Being overweight also increases your risk of heart disease in several other ways. Everyone in this country is more likely to die of a heart attack than anything else and the more overweight you are, the more your risk of heart disease increases. For men aged 35–44 years, it has been shown that a 10 per cent increase in weight increases the chance of heart disease by 38 per cent. A 20 per cent increase in weight pushes up the risk of a heart attack by 86 per cent. Women are not immune from this effect, although in this age group their risk of heart disease is less than men's. This protective effect is thought to be caused by female sex hormones. The difference does disappear after the menopause.

Overweight and high blood pressure

Being even slightly overweight can cause a rise in blood pressure and for some susceptible people it will be quite a serious rise. High blood pressure increases the chance of heart attacks and strokes but losing weight often has the beneficial effect of returning blood pressure to normal. Indeed, doctors often advise patients with high blood pressure to try to lose some weight as their blood pressure may then return to normal without the need to take any medication.

Overweight and diabetes

There are two types of diabetes: one that can occur in young people and needs injections of insulin to treat it and another that begins in middle or old age and can be treated by tablets or diet or both. This latter type is caused by being overweight, and the risk of developing diabetes increases with the degree of obesity.

Overweight and gall-stones

The fatter you are, the more likely you are to develop stones in your gall bladder. This is due to the greater amount of cholesterol that fat people tend to have: the cholesterol is precipitated out of the bile to form stones.

Another factor which makes gall-stones more likely in fat people is the use of inappropriate and outdated slimming diets such as low carbohydrate or low-fibre diets which tend to encourage the formation of gall-stones.

Overweight and cancer

Statistically there are greater risks of developing certain types of cancer in those who are overweight. In men, there's a greater chance of developing cancer of the colon, the rectum and the prostate. In women, the likelihood of developing cancer of the breast, womb and cervix is increased. All of these are quite common cancers and there's also an increased risk of developing some less common ones such as cancer of the gall bladder.

Overweight and lung disease

One of the commonest complaints of those who are overweight is breathlessness on mild exertion, such as walking uphill or upstairs. Various measurements of the lungs' ability to function properly show that their capacity deteriorates as obesity develops. If you're overweight, you're more likely to develop a chest infection after having an operation.

Overweight and arthritis

The most common form of arthritis is osteoarthritis which tends to affect everyone as they get older as it's a mechanical effect of the joints wearing out. This form of arthritis improves after losing weight.

Gout is a rarer form of arthritis, the risk of which increases in men who are very overweight.

Overweight and varicose veins

In those who are obese, or severely overweight (that is, 20 per cent above their ideal weight), the risk of developing varicose veins doubles.

Overweight and irregular periods

Being overweight can lead to various menstrual abnormalities and being severely overweight can cause heavy and painful periods. The hormonal imbalance that is caused by being overweight can also lead to the distressing symptom of hirsutism: an increase and change in the normal distribution of body hair.

Overweight and feeling tired and weary

Feeling tired may not sound as serious as some of the other complications of being overweight, but it can be quite debilitating and seriously diminish the quality of life. It's not a surprising symptom: if you're a couple of stone overweight, it's as if you're carrying around a couple of heavy suitcases all the time. This excess weight will also probably give you backache and make a slipped disc more likely.

Overweight and mental health

Being fat isn't just a matter of illness and getting slim isn't just a matter of physical health. For some people, being fat and wanting to be slim is the most important thing in their life. Being fat can make them so unhappy that they start overeating for comfort which, like a vicious spiral, just makes them fatter still.

If being fat is getting you depressed or if you know you're indulging in huge binges, you need professional help. It's important for you to see your GP.

Whatever your reasons for wanting to lose weight – and they may be very important – one compelling reason, as you've seen, is that you will improve your health and decrease the risks of developing a wide range of diseases.

3 Why am I Fat?

How is it that you, who desperately nibble at lettuce leaves and low-fat cottage cheese, are fat while your friend, who gorges on chips, chocolate and cream cakes, is thin? It's unfair, yes: life is unfair in this as in so many other ways. This chapter explains why some of us are fat and some are thin – not only individuals but whole nations. Once you understand why your body is the way it is, you've got the knowledge and therefore the power to do something about it. You can't change the person you are, but you need only be a product not a prisoner of your genes.

A NATION OF FATTIES

Since the end of the Second World War there's been a progressive increase in the average weight for height of adults in the United Kingdom. Unfortunately this hasn't been due to an increase in healthy muscle: over that time the average amount of body fat in adults has gone up by 10 per cent. Remember that's an average: it is not evenly spread and those millions of pounds of excess fat are found on the *half* of the population which is overweight. It's because we've become less active, and have been taking in too much fatty, sugary food for the amount of work we do. In the recent past, our forebears may have eaten *more* calories than we do, but because they were so physically active, they burnt them off and so were less likely to get fat.

OBESITY: THE WESTERN EPIDEMIC

Looking at what happens to whole populations over decades is very useful for understanding health and disease. One of the biggest puzzles in medical science is why some people get infections or diseases and others don't. Before vaccinations rendered the disease so rare, not everyone exposed to the polio virus developed polio. In the middle ages, the Bubonic Plague, known as the Black Death, wiped out at least a quarter of the population of Europe but it didn't kill everyone. Why? We're here to tell the tale and ask the question.

The best modern example of a killer disease is the epidemic of our own century: heart disease. This was very rare until 50 or 60 years ago and its prevalence now can only be explained by understanding that the whole population has changed its behaviour by, for example, smoking more, exercising less and eating more fat. That doesn't mean that *everyone* will have a heart attack, but it does mean that where the behaviour which increases the risk of heart disease is common, then very many people in the population will develop it. They are the people who are 'susceptible'; the majority, it seems, in the case of heart disease. The same thing is seen if we look at the incidence of high blood pressure: most people eat a high salt diet in this country and for some that can help to cause high blood pressure. Others can eat a lot of salt without any effect on their blood pressure. Therefore if the *average* level of salt eaten in the country came down, then the number of people suffering from high blood pressure – the 'incidence' of the disease – would also be reduced.

This is a difficult concept but an extremely important one. If the whole population changed its lifestyle in certain key respects, heart disease would no longer be a mass killer. But if everyone had reduced their risk of a heart attack to the absolute minimum, a *small* number of people would still get heart disease, and they are fated to get it no matter what they do. *Most* of us, though, are in charge of our own destiny in this respect.

The same applies to the problem of being overweight. In our present society it's a mass problem affecting about half of the population and, perhaps even two-thirds or more of us are susceptible to some degree of weight gain.

But although this is true throughout the affluent West, it is not the case for all populations. The vast majority of people in India or China live a rural, peasant lifestyle and their diet consists largely of rice, pulses and vegetables with very little meat. Most of them are involved in manual labour and very, very few of them are overweight. Of course there are *some* people in those countries who are: either those who are following a more Westernised lifestyle and diet or those who belong to the 'irreducible minimum'. In the case of being overweight, these are people who have glandular or metabolic illnesses which account for their obesity.

These illnesses are very rare: they account for 5 per cent or less of the people in the United Kingdom who are very overweight (20 per cent or more over their ideal weight). So for the majority of us who are overweight it's our lifestyle which has 'brought out' this hidden susceptibility to fatness.

FAT BABIES BECOME FAT ADULTS

There is some evidence that the way we are fed in infancy and childhood may have long-term effects. In fact, it has been suggested that the increase in weight of young adults in the 1980s reflects inappropriate infant feeding in the 1950s and 1960s. It has been demonstrated that bottle-fed babies are particularly likely to show an excessive weight gain. Of course, with babies, unlike adults, it used to be said that 'big is beautiful'; babies were never fat, only 'bonny'. Babies who are fat are more likely to turn into children who are fat who, in turn, are more likely to grow into adults who are fat. It's not inevitable that all fat babies and children will grow into fat adults, but it's more likely. So we need to keep an eye on our children's weight as well as our own.

About 7 per cent of pre-teenage children are overweight and the problem increases as children get older. Half of British 20-year-olds are already at the upper limit of their ideal weight or going over it. By the age of 25, 31 per cent of men and 27 per cent of women are substantially overweight – that is, more than 10 per cent above their desirable weight and so at risk of ill-health.

SO WHY AM I FAT?

Are we programmed to be fat, then? Should we be fatalistic and decide to be fat but happy? In fact, like so many other characteristics - our height, our intelligence, our personality - being overweight or slim is determined by a combination of the characteristics which we inherit from our parents and the circumstances in which we live. Some of us (very few) are programmed to be fat; some of us (in fact, most of us) are programmed to be fat or thin depending on the sort of life we live; and the lucky others are programmed to be thin no matter what they do.

THE FOUR THINGS THAT DETERMINE OUR WEIGHT

There are four things that determine whether or not we are fat. Two of them we can decisively influence:

* How much food we eat.

* How much exercise and physical activity we undertake.

The other two are programmed into our bodies, but there is some evidence that we can influence them, at least a little:

* Our basal metabolic rate (BMR), that is, the 'tickover' speed of our body's functioning.

* Our rate of thermogenesis, or the ability of the body to burn up excess calories as heat.

How much food do we eat?

This is, of course, one of the decisive factors in whether or not we become overweight. But it's important to note that 'how much' doesn't mean how much in weight or quantity, but how much in terms of calories or food energy. In these terms, 1 lb of chocolate is *more* than 10 lb of apples because it contains more calories. But in terms of a satisfying quantity, the apples, of course, are 'more'. Herein is the key to successful - and painless - weight loss. We can eat our fill of many foods and still lose weight. This is the principle behind the success of *The BBC Diet* (see chapter 5).

How much physical activity do we do?

It's really been a shock to medical researchers to discover how few calories many people burn up over and above the energy needed just to keep our body going. Our forebears could accuse us not so much of the sin of gluttony but of sloth. See p. 360 for ideas on how to increase your everyday activity.

You may feel you take just as much exercise as some of your thin friends, but, unfortunately, their bodies may be much better than yours at burning up calories. That's not disastrous for you: it just means you have to try a little harder!

Our basal metabolic rate (BMR)

As I've said, this is the 'tickover' speed of the body; the rate at which it uses up energy just to keep its essential functions going, like the heart beating, our lungs expanding and contracting, and our temperature at the correct level. This does vary from person to person. It's those people with a lower BMR who are more at risk of becoming overweight. There are two things about our BMR that you need to know:

* When we start to diet, our BMR may go *down* a little as the body tries to conserve energy (after all, it thought it was laying down all that fat for a possible future famine, and it tries to keep it). This is one of the reasons why really drastic crash diets are a bad idea. Apart from being dangerous, they tend to push down our BMR and so are not even more effective anyway. There's more about this aspect of the BMR going down on a diet, and what can be done about it, in chapter 21.

* Our BMR *increases* in response to increased physical activity. That's why it's so important to try to increase your activity if you want to lose weight most effectively (again, this is discussed further in chapter 21).

Thermogenesis

This is the body's ability to burn off excess calories as heat and it varies from person to person. We don't know everything about this process and a lot more research work needs to be done on it, but thermogenesis seems to occur partly in response to eating food and its rate may depend on the *type* of food eaten. There's some evidence now that calories may be burned up more slowly on a high-fat diet. Experiments with animals seem to indicate that high-fat diets encourage weight gain. By following the low-fat BBC

Diet you'll not only be reducing the number of calories you eat, but may also be burning up those calories you do eat more efficiently.

Experimental evidence also shows that diet-induced thermogenesis may be increased by taking exercise. This is in addition to both the higher BMR induced by exercise and to the calories the exercise itself burns off. With this double whammy attack, *The BBC Diet* gives you the very best way to lose those excess pounds.

4 A Dozen Dieting Myths

MYTH 1: DIFFERENT COMBINATIONS OF FOOD CAN HELP YOU BURN UP FAT

This myth has been around a long time with pineapple diets, papaya diets, grapefruit diets and Bai-lin tea diets! The idea put forward is that each of these things has a magic ingredient or secret enzyme, previously unknown to medical science, and recently and miraculously discovered. Eat the magic ingredient and then you can eat what you like: gallons of ice-cream, pounds of chocolate, lashings of butter. All your excess fat will be burnt up and your life will be transformed for ever with no effort from you whatsoever. Baloney!

I'm not saying that some of these diets won't help you to lose some weight: it's possible they will, but there's no magic about it. If you try to follow the sort of diet that says 'eat dozens of grapefruit a day' or 'eat as much pineapple a day as you want', or even the sort that says 'first eat a dozen papayas a day – and then anything you like', you may lose some weight. (If you did eat as many grapefruit as you wanted but nothing else, you'd certainly lose weight: you'd have to eat 12 lb of grapefruit before you reached 1000 calories!)

These types of diet are just a way of cutting calories – the hard way. If you do just stick to one or two foods like this, you can't help but cut calories and so lose weight but it's difficult, abnormal, boring and a con – and certainly isn't an effective way of *continuing* to lose weight.

One- or two-food diets can be dangerous (your body needs nutrients other than calories) and, of course, you won't learn anything from these diets about the way you were eating before which caused you to get fat in the first place.

As for the 'drink half a cup of Bai-lin tea and then eat anything else you like' type of diets, which don't even suggest cutting calories . . . well, ask yourself honestly if you really believe them. If there was a magic ingredient that would keep us all trim and healthy, don't you think they'd be putting it in the water?!

MYTH 2: THE AMOUNT OF ALCOHOL YOU DRINK DOESN'T REALLY AFFECT YOUR WEIGHT

It surprises me, but many people really do believe that it's only food which makes them put on weight. Because alcoholic drinks are not food, then somehow they don't count. Or people sometimes think that drinks that are not sweet – like a pint of bitter or dry white wine – don't contain any calories.

In fact, alcoholic drink contains calories not only in the form of sugar (which varies depending on the type of drink) but also in the pure alcohol contained in the drink as well – and that pure alcohol is high in calories. Booze can be a significant factor in determining whether or not we are overweight.

One contestant on the BBC television series *Go For It* two or three years ago, 29-year-old Simon Payne, was drinking about 8 pints of beer a day when the series began. He was 5′ 10″ tall and weighed 22 stone and 10 lb. And no wonder – those 8 pints of beer a day were clocking up about 12 000 calories a week! Simon cut his drinking right down and in less than 2 months lost 3 stone.

The average person in this country gets about 10 per cent of daily calories from alcoholic drinks – that's drinking 2 or 3 drinks a day. It's important to remember that alcohol supplies us with no nutrients and so in that sense they're 'empty' calories. You don't need to cut out drink completely if you want to lose weight, but if you're drinking a lot you do need to cut it right down.

Approximately 1 glass of wine or ½ pint of beer, lager or cider or 1 glass of sherry, port or martini or 1 single pub measure of spirits like gin or whisky with a mixer, each contains about 100 calories. (Each of these measures also contains 1 unit of alcohol, and for your health's sake you should drink fewer than 21 units of alcohol a week if you're a man and fewer than 14 units if you're a woman.)

MYTH 3: 'WE'RE ALL BIG IN OUR FAMILY AND, ANYWAY, I DON'T EAT ENOUGH TO KEEP A SPARROW ALIVE'

It's true that being overweight *seems* to run in families: in any supermarket you can see overweight parents dragging around their equally overweight children. But look at what's in the shopping trolley: biscuits, cakes, meat pies, sausages, chocolate. If those children had been brought up with low-fat yoghurt and fresh fruit and grilled fish, would they be overweight? What certainly does run in families is the view of what constitutes a 'normal' diet.

But 'we're all big in our family' is no reason for *you* to be overweight. What we probably do inherit from our parents are things like the tickover speed of our body's machine (our BMR, see p. 40) and the way our body handles food and burns it up. There is, of course, a variation in this: some people can eat enormous quantities and not put on weight.

'I don't eat enough to keep a sparrow alive' was a cry I

often used to hear when I was in general practice. It does seem unfair that you don't seem to eat very much and others eat so much more and don't put on weight. But if you are overweight, what is indisputable is that you're eating too much for the way your body is built and the activity you undertake; and you're probably eating smallish quantities of food packed with fat and sugar, like cakes and biscuits. You could eat *more* food and feel satisfied and eat *fewer* calories. You also need to start exercising more – even if it's only walking.

It is true that people can be very overweight, have a low BMR and not seem to eat or need huge amounts of food. It's more difficult for you to lose weight and you'll need more patience, but it's not impossible. Following *The BBC Diet*'s guidelines of less fat and sugar, but more fibre and exercise is exactly what you need. Never lose sight of the fact that every excess ounce didn't appear out of nowhere, but went in by your mouth at some time. And you can get rid of it.

MYTH 4: 'ON SOME DIETS YOU CAN LOSE 20 LB IN 2 WEEKS'

20 lb of what? It can't be fat – that's a scientific impossibility as your body just can't get rid of such an amount of fat in such a short time.

There's a difference between losing weight and losing fat. You could lose *weight* – say 7 lb or so – in a Turkish bath by sweating it out in a few hours. But you wouldn't have lost any *fat* at all: as soon as you have something to drink, the weight goes back on again as your body rehydrates. The key to sustained weight loss is losing fat.

On any diet which cuts calories sufficiently, you will get a rapid weight loss in the first couple of weeks. This will happen on *The BBC Diet*. But I certainly don't claim that it is *all* fat that you have lost.

Quite a lot of the weight you lose at the beginning of a diet is water: but it's different from the water you might sweat out in a Turkish bath and you don't put the weight back on if you drink a couple of pints of water. The water you will lose at the start of a diet is bound up with glycogen in our muscles and the liver. Glycogen is the way the body stores sugar – in fact, it's just glucose molecules stuck together with water. It's a more immediate energy store for the body than fat is, and so when we start to diet, our body uses up this immediate store first before it gets to work on the fat.

This is true of all diets, despite those extravagant claims to the contrary. The body doesn't start to burn up fat straight away. Most of that initial, fast weight loss is not fat. But that's not to say we should dismiss it: it's certainly some weight lost and it should be a good morale boost at the beginning of a diet. And, of course, it's preparing the body to get down to the real business of burning up fat.

But that burning up of fat is a slower process, which is why our weight loss slows down after the first early phase lasting a couple of weeks. There's no way round this and it's something you should be prepared for so you aren't disappointed and discouraged. But if you carry on with your diet, you will continue to lose weight – and more importantly, fat – at a steady rate and you will *keep it off*. See chapter 23 for how much weight you can lose and how quickly you can realistically expect to lose it.

MYTH 5: 'SOME DIETS CAN GET RID OF THE FAT JUST IN THE PLACES YOU WANT TO LOSE IT'

Wouldn't it be wonderful if we could lose weight selectively from just the bits of the body we wanted? Like aiming a ray gun and getting rid of our double chin or our thunder thighs or our beer belly? It'd speed up the whole process, too!

Unfortunately, fat is fat is fat and when we start taking in fewer calories than our body needs for the activity we do, it starts burning up the fat from *all* the fat stores of the body, and so the places where most fat is stored – like our paunch or our hips – are the last bits to go. There's no way of directing the body so that it takes 'a bit more off here, but not so much off there'.

There are two things you *can* do though. First of all: don't be tempted to go on a crash diet. It's on these sort of diets that the fat suddenly seems to fall off your face before the rest of the body has caught up!

Secondly, start taking some exercise. General exercise, like walking or swimming, tones up all the muscles in your body and so you're going to start looking in better shape as your muscles become firmer. And there are some exercises you can do which will help to tone up different muscle groups – such as those in your hips and thighs – so that the disappearing fat is replaced by healthy-looking firmer flesh (see chapter 21).

MYTH 6: 'YOU ALWAYS NEED TO COUNT EVERY SINGLE CALORIE TO LOSE WEIGHT EFFECTIVELY'

It's possible to become a little obsessive when you're going on a diet, thinking 'I'd better have this apple rather than that one because it looks a bit smaller'. Go ahead and have two apples. It's only 40 calories more than one, and believe me two apples have a great deal of filling power, so you'll automatically be forced to cut down more somewhere else. Of course, I couldn't say that if it were slices of chocolate gâteau you were counting!

We really need only concern ourselves with calories in their hundreds. You don't need to count calories to lose weight effectively, but you do need to know some guidelines so that you have a developed 'calorie-awareness'. To fret about single calories is crazy: four peas, two baked beans and two slices of cucumber all contain 1 calorie – ½ oz (15 g) of butter, on the other hand, contains 100! So it is important to know which kinds of food are packed with calories and which aren't (see chapter 5). It's much better to have this *understanding* rather than relying on calorie charts, and if you do put this knowledge into practice, you'll automatically cut calories without having to count them.

MYTH 7: 'YOU'VE GOT TO GO HUNGRY IF YOU'RE REALLY GOING TO LOSE WEIGHT'

The caricature image of a dieter is someone who nibbles lettuce leaves and whose day's highlight is a crispbread spread with a very thin smear of cottage cheese.

How puritanical we are! There's almost a feeling that we have to be punished for being overweight, that we have to expiate our guilt by half-starving! A variation of this idea is that all 'slimming' food has to be nasty – the medicine has to taste unpleasant before it's doing you any good.

All this is based on a fundamentally mistaken notion of why most people get overweight. It's not that they're gorging nightly on fresh cream slices – it's simply that, without realising it, they are taking in large quantities of fat and sugar in their everyday food. It's not the occasional sinful treats that make us fat, but what we take in, day after day, year after year as ordinary sustenance. Often it's the food we hardly think about that makes us fat, and not the food that we particularly enjoy as a sporadic indulgence.

If we understand where fat, sugar and fibre lurk (see chapter 9) and follow *The BBC Diet*, we really can eat our fill, enjoy our food and lose weight. It isn't a conjuring trick or a riddle – it's understanding and putting into practice that crucial difference between quantity of food and the concentration of calories in food, and once you've understood it, it can transform your life!

MYTH 8: 'YOU HAVE TO STICK
TO A DIET TO THE LETTER'

A lady wrote to me last year, as she was following *The BBC Diet*, and asked 'on the last day, it says I should have cabbage. I don't like cabbage, so can I just miss it out or will this stop the fat from being burnt up?' This took me back a bit, as I thought I had explained very clearly that it was what you *didn't* eat that would make you lose weight and not what you *did*.

The lady was obviously subscribing to the seemingly widely-held view that there is a mystical formula of food which, when eaten in a certain order, will spirit away the fat. Needless to say, there isn't. Diets aren't designed – the BBC one isn't, anyway! – so that the combination of ingredients somehow creates powerful magic. I can't stress enough that, when it comes down to it, losing weight (the concept, at least) is really very simple: you just have to take in fewer calories than your body burns up and so force it to start burning up the fat. So you avoid calorie-rich foods like fat and sugar and you eat more foods which are relatively low in calories (like those high in fibres).

I understand, of course, that some people want a clear plan in front of them, with the quantities worked out, so they know they're doing everything 'right'. This is fine, and you can of course follow one of the plans to the letter if you prefer to. But please don't think of it as some religious rite which has to be stuck to rigidly in order for its magic to work for you.

Our weight isn't controlled by dark and mysterious forces that we have to appease! You can *understand* why you've put on weight; you can *understand* the principles behind losing it. I want you to understand *The BBC Diet*, and not follow it blindly for two reasons: firstly, you'll never again be at the mercy of quacks and charlatans (particularly if they want to relieve you of a tidy sum of money for losing weight); secondly, you will take the principles with you for ever – and that knowledge will give you power, over your weight and your health.

MYTH 9: 'THE BEST WAY TO LOSE WEIGHT IS TO FORGET ABOUT FOOD FOR A COUPLE OF WEEKS AND JUST TAKE THOSE FUNNY CHEMICAL DRINKS'

The 'funny chemical drinks' are of course those fashionable but expensive concoctions – 'very low-calorie diets' (or VLCDs). You don't need to think about food at all with them, but just mix the sachet of chemicals with water and use them to replace meals.

Again, I think they appeal to puritanism: food is evil, overweight is an illness, therefore let's take this nasty medicine. I think they also appeal to a sense of helplessness: 'I really can't lose weight myself as I have no willpower, therefore I shall just put myself in the hands of the inventors of these sachets'.

There are two things to be said about VLCDs. First of all, they are a waste of money for, as a British government medical committee has reported 'there is no evidence that VLCD regimes are more likely to achieve enduring weight loss than conventional weight-reducing diets'. Second, they do nothing at all to help you understand why you got fat in the first place. You may lose weight on them, but you have done nothing to change those fattening eating habits – so of course you're going to put on weight again.

Isn't there something unpleasant, too, about exchanging real food for this set of chemicals? And following one of these regimes not only cuts you off from the pleasure of food, but also cuts you off from family and friends sharing mealtimes with you – you're in a corner, sipping your chemicals!

MYTH 10: 'STARVATION IS THE MOST EFFEC-TIVE WAY TO GET THIN!'

This is, superficially, a seductive idea. Why bother at all with what you can or can't eat on a diet? Why not just starve yourself for a few days, particularly if you want to get into a bikini and that Greek beach is beckoning next week?

Starving yourself is, of course, extremely dangerous. Although some people have survived many weeks without food, there are cases of people dying, suddenly and unexpectedly, after starving themselves for only a few days. This happens because of the quick and unpredictable upsets in the chemical balance in the body.

And, in fact, total starvation is not a particularly spectacular way to lose weight. After the rapid initial weight-loss phase, people who have starved themselves completely lose weight only at the rate of about 4 lb (1.75 kg) a week. The body by that time, of course, is really closing things down and desperately trying to conserve its fat stores and stay alive.

Also, the weight loss which happens in conditions of total starvation is highly undesirable. About half the weight lost is not *fat* at all, but *lean* tissue; the body starts burning up its own muscles. By comparison, of the weight lost on a diet of 1000 calories, three-quarters is fat and only a quarter is lean tissue. This is why drastic crash diets just make no sense whatsoever: you're engaged in a struggle with your body which you can't win. The more severe the diet, the more desperately the body tries to hang on to every ounce of fat. The softly-softly approach wins hands down every time!

MYTH 11: 'EXERCISE DOESN'T HAVE ANY EFFECT ON WEIGHT LOSS'

It's true that it would take a brisk three-quarters of an hour walk to burn off the calories from a slice of chocolate cake (though, to me that seems a fair exchange!) but that's not the end of the story.

Over a period of time, even small changes to our everyday life – and I'm not talking about formal 'exercise' – can burn up the calories and make a significant difference to our weight. (There's a list of suggestions for 'small changes' in chapter 21.)

But more physical activity is also important for slimmers for the effect it seems to have on our body's tickover speed or BMR (see p. 40). Going on any diet tends to reduce our BMR – our rate of burning up calories while the body is 'at rest' – by a little. Regular exercise seems to counter this effect and so enables us to burn up calories more efficiently – not just during the period when we are exercising, but during the rest of the time too, when we're sitting watching television, for example! It also tends to increase our body's ability to burn up any excess calories (by thermogenesis, see p. 40).

You can lose weight of course, just by cutting down the calories you take in. You can also lose weight by just increasing the amount of physical activity you undertake. But the most efficient and effective way to lose weight is to do a combination of the two – and this is exactly what *The BBC Diet* suggests.

MYTH 12: 'YOU'RE HEALTHIER THE WAY NATURE INTENDED YOU TO BE – AND IF THAT'S FAT, SO BE IT!'

If you're just 'pleasantly plump', your excess weight probably isn't having any effect on your health – though even losing half a stone or so may reduce the level of cholesterol in your blood or bring down your blood pressure if it's high.

But by the time you start getting more than 20 per cent or so above your desirable weight (12 stone instead of 10 stone, say) then you start to increase the risk of a range of diseases. Being overweight can push up the level of fats, including cholesterol, in your blood and it can increase your blood pressure: in turn, these can increase your risk of a heart attack.

Being overweight can lead to diabetes, gall-stones, varicose veins; it can exacerbate arthritis and back problems; and of course it can just make you feel weary and tired all the time (see chapter 2).

Losing weight can improve your health in many hidden ways, and it can also reduce risks you didn't even know you were running.

But, of course, most people who are fat and who lose weight say how much better they actually feel: they have more energy and more zest for life. Many people who lose weight say they feel so much more confident, or they feel younger, or they take up new hobbies and interests. They feel like different people. Now, no matter what nature 'intended', that's worth going for!

5 A Friend and Two Foes

If you want to lose weight, your friend is fibre and your two foes are fat and sugar. Fashions in dieting have swung about all over the place in the last 10 or 15 years, with low-carbohydrate diets, high-protein diets and high-fibre diets. Some of these have been based more on the whim of the inventors than on any scientific evidence. But the chemical properties of fibre, fat and sugar are unchanging and unchangeable. There are many ways to lose weight but the easiest, most effective and healthiest is by following a diet which cuts fat and sugar and increases fibre. That's the best way to cut calories without feeling hungry and so it's the most surefire way to slim. It's *The BBC Diet* way!

'FATTENERS' VERSUS 'FILLERS'

There is no mystery about this 'friend and two foes' way of dieting. When you want to lose weight, there are four basic principles to remember:

* You have to carry on eating (trying to starve is a bad idea and a bad way of trying to lose fat, see p. 51).

* You want to feel full and satisfied with the food you eat so you're not tempted to binge.

* You need food which fills you but doesn't contain too many calories.

* You need to avoid food which doesn't particularly fill you and is packed with calories.

The basic properties of fibre, fat and sugar explain why one is a friend and two are foes!

Weight-for-weight, fibre doesn't contain too many calories. When you eat fibre-rich foods, you tend to get full before you can take in too many calories. That's why these foods are described as filling not fattening.

Both fat and sugar pack many calories into a small space – they're so lacking in bulk. So with these foods you can eat far too many calories before you get full. Weight-for-weight, pure fat contains *twice* as many calories as pure protein or pure carbohydrate. In practice, of course, most food is a mixture of all three (and water) in varying proportions but when fat is present in significant amounts the calorie count starts shooting up. In nature, sugar invariably comes bound up with fibre, as in fresh fruit, which limits the amount of it you can eat. However, once processed and unnaturally concentrated, it is packed with calories. Just look at some comparisons:

* 2 teaspoons of sugar contain as many calories as 4 oz (100 g) of peas. Does a cup of tea with two sugars 'fill you up' in the way a quarter of a pound of peas would help to? No.

* 1 oz (25 g) of butter (which is almost pure fat) contains *more* calories than 10 oz (275 g) of potatoes (which are mostly digestible carbohydrate bulked out with fibre and water). Now 10 oz (275 g) of potatoes is really quite a large helping – it would certainly fill me up! But an ounce of butter could be scoffed, melted on half a potato, without even batting an eyelid.

* 10 lb (4.5 kg) of apples contain *fewer* calories than 1 lb (450 g) of chocolates. So you could eat a whole pound of apples for the same number of calories as a couple of

chocolates! The reason is that chocolate packs a huge punch of fat and sugar into a small space. Could you eat much else after a pound of apples? A couple of chocolates could be gone in a blink!

These comparisons are good news, of course, for people who want to lose weight. Because if you choose the *right* foods you will eat your fill, not feel hungry and certainly lose weight! That's the key to the success of *The BBC Diet*.

WHY THE AVERAGE BRITISH DIET MAKES US FAT

As we've already seen, our problem is that our lifestyles are becoming so inactive that we're consuming excessive calories for our way of life.

When we consider our health, as we've seen, it's not only the number of calories that is important, it is also where these calories are coming from. Since the beginning of this century our diet has changed so that we now eat more fat and less 'complex' carbohydrates – like the starches and fibre found in fruit, vegetables and cereals – and we're now eating vastly more sugar. The amount of protein we eat has remained about the same.

Some of these changes have happened because we have more money to spend on food and some foods have become relatively much cheaper. Fashion, and different views of what's healthy, have also played their part in altering the pattern of the food we eat. But some of the most important changes have happened because of the way much of the food is now sold to us. We're now eating a lot of food which may not have been touched by human hand but has certainly been touched by a great deal of machinery – processed food.

Processing food – refining it, taking things out of it, putting other things into it, mixing it together and packaging it – has often meant making it cheaper. Sometimes it's made it more nutritious too, though not always.

For example, when the machine milling of rice was introduced in the Far East, it was considered a great advance and people found the resulting polished rice, with the husk taken off, much more palatable. But an important vitamin, B_1 or thiamine, is present in significant amounts in the outer husk and for people living on a rice-based diet this is an important source of the vitamin. By eating the polished rice, now lacking in B_1, they began to get the disease beri-beri.

This story illustrates how our bodies may sometimes be tricked. Polished rice tasted as good as whole rice and there was nothing to show that it was lacking something – until people became ill.

This is one of the problems with processed foods: they may be lacking some of the nutrients that whole, unrefined 'natural' foods supply, as I explain below. (Though it should be said that some processed foods have nutrients added to them; for example, vitamins are added by law to margarine.) There's also another aspect to processed foods of particular concern to those who want to lose weight.

The problem is the opposite of a lack of nutrients – it's a surfeit of calories. Processing food can cause large numbers of calories to be packed into a small space, because it so often includes those two 'calorie-packers': fat and sugar. Take the case of the 10 lb (4.5 kg) of apples having fewer calories than 1 lb (450 g) of chocolates. Whole, natural, unrefined food like an apple has a low calorie-to-weight ratio, or low energy-density because it's packed with fibre and water. It's impossible to take in too many calories by eating this type of food, because before we have done so, we feel full and satisfied. But refined foods often have a very high calorie-to-weight ratio, or high energy-density, and so we can, weight for weight, eat far more and therefore take in a large number of calories before we feel full.

As already noted, fat and sugar are the two culprits in making processed food energy-dense and, like the terrible twins, they often make an appearance together. Chocolate, for example, is largely sweetened fat. A large quantity of the products of the food industry rely on sweetening fat, as in chocolate biscuits and cakes, or on salting it, as in crisps, sausages, pies and pasties, in order to make it palatable. If we were eating unprocessed food that we could recognise we wouldn't possibly eat so much fat. A meat pie or sausage may deliver half or more of its large dose of calories in fat. Fat is cheaper than meat, so it's mixed with meat and other things in order to become palatable and to make us buy it.

There's another twist to this story, which is important for everyone's health whether or not they need to lose weight. We don't rely on our food just for calories or energy but also for nutrients, for minerals, for vitamins, for essential amino acids – all substances that our body can't manufacture. As our food has become high in energy-density, it's also become low in nutrient-density. This is going to be an increasing danger in the future. If our intake of calories falls, as our physical activity reduces, we may be in danger of not getting enough nutrients from the food we eat. Calorie for calorie we get less nutrients from processed food with high energy-density than we do from natural wholefood with low energy-density. By 'natural wholefood', I don't mean food from health shops; you can buy natural wholefood in any supermarket. It's food you can recognise immediately and see what plant or tree it grew on or what fish or animal it came from.

So although we may be taking in enough calories – or too many – we may still be malnourished if our food isn't sufficiently rich with the nutrients we need.

This is the danger of some diets which cut down the calories but also cut down valuable nutrients. However, the balanced and healthy BBC Diet avoids this and, even though you're cutting down the calories, you should be increasing the nutrients by following our guidelines.

Now let's look at our friend and foes in more detail.

FIBRE

Fibre is now firmly fixed in most people's minds as 'good'. Dieters tend to have more ambiguous feelings about the word 'carbohydrate' but, in fact, fibre *is* carbohydrate. There was a confusion in yesterday's diets which lumped together all carbohydrates as 'fattening'. Although sugar is also a carbohydrate and certainly is fattening, it's what's called a 'simple' carbohydrate – that means it's certainly 'pure' as its manufacturers claim. It's pure because it contains nothing else, it's concentrated and packed with calories. Every grain of sugar we take is converted into energy (or fat!) by our body. Fibre, on the other hand, is what's called a 'complex' carbohydrate, as are the starchy carbohydrates found in potatoes and bread. Complex carbohydrates normally come bulked out with water and so help to fill us up. Fibre is also described as 'unavailable' carbohydrate: our stomachs can't digest it. So, although it helps to fill us up, it passes straight through us!

Lumping all carbohydrates together has caused a confusion in some people's minds: 'surely', they say, 'bread and potatoes are fattening?' The truth is they are not: they're so filling and satisfying, that we feel full before we take in 'danger levels' of calories. They *do* become fattening, though, when we start adding fat to them: frying potatoes as chips or spreading butter on the bread. Then the calorie count goes right up. But, as *The BBC Diet* shows, there are many ways of enjoying these foods without adding all those surplus calories.

A good intake of fibre is incorporated into *The BBC Diet* and if you want to follow it flexibly and follow its guidelines without choosing a particular diet plan, see chapter 9 for ways of increasing the amount of fibre you eat.

How fibre helps with weight loss

As I've explained, the most important way fibre helps with weight loss is by satisfying our hunger so that we're not tempted to eat fatty and sugary foods. Fibre-rich foods take longer to chew and when they reach the stomach, they absorb some water and these two things help increase the feeling of fullness. (This is why it is important to drink plenty of water when you increase your fibre intake – always have a glass of mineral or tap water with each meal.) Fibre is our friend against those foes: fat and sugar.

Remember the three Fs:

FIBRE: FILLING not FATTENING

However, fibre also helps us to lose weight in two other ways:

* Fibre-rich foods help to slow down the rate at which our bodies absorb sugar from food into the bloodstream. This is important because if we have a meal high in sugar, our body reacts by pouring out the hormone insulin into the blood. This hormone regulates the level of sugar in the blood, and a surge of it after a high sugar meal can push the level of sugar in the blood right down. This causes us to feel hunger between meals. When we eat lots of fibre-rich food, the levels of blood sugar tend to be more steady and to fluctuate less.

* Because our stomachs can't break down fibre, it passes straight through our digestive system (helping the whole process, incidentally). There's now some evidence that fibre-rich foods may help to reduce the amount of energy, the number of calories, that our bodies can extract from food.

Are there any drawbacks to fibre?

Like all friends, fibre may have one or two characteristics that we're not too keen on!

Very large amounts of fibre may interfere with the absorption of some minerals that we need – in particular, iron and calcium. But you have to go really over the top with fibre for this to be a problem. By following *The BBC Diet*, you are nowhere near increasing your fibre to the levels where this could be a problem. Also, you'll be getting enough iron and calcium anyway. Iron is found in meat, liver, peas, beans and dark green vegetables, and if you are eating plenty of fresh fruit and vegetables, the vitamin C in these helps your body to absorb the iron it needs.

Calcium is found in milk and in fact skimmed milk has a higher proportion of calcium in it than whole milk. Yoghurt, fish, bread and dark green vegetables are also good sources of calcium.

Some fibre-rich foods, particularly pulses, peas and beans, can cause gas in the intestines. (Our intestines normally produce about a couple of pints of gas a day.) Some people find that they do get problems with wind when they start increasing fibre in their diet. Most find that, as their body adapts to the extra fibre, this problem disappears of its own accord. If it is a problem for you, reduce the amount of peas and beans you eat and then reintroduce them gradually. If you are cooking dried peas or beans, throw away the soaking water and boil them in fresh. Gas should only be a temporary problem but, if it is a nuisance for you, remember that there are many sources of fibre other than peas and beans that will not cause a gas problem (see pp. 105–6).

Fibre and health

One of the problems with the average British diet is that we're not eating enough fibre. Apart from the serious

61

medical conditions associated with a low-fibre diet which are outlined below, this lack of fibre leaves us with room in our tummies for those fatty sugary foods which make us overweight. The average British diet at the moment contains just under ½ oz (15 g) of fibre a day. This is very low compared with, for example, rural Africans whose intake is between 2 and 4½ oz (50 and 120 g) of fibre a day. During the Second World War, 1¼ to 1½ oz (32–40 g) of fibre a day was the average intake and at present vegetarians in the UK consume 1½ oz (40 g) a day on average. The consensus of medical opinion is that we should be eating at least 1¼ oz (32 g) of fibre a day – at least double our present average intake. You'll be doing this on *The BBC Diet* and losing weight.

Many diseases which are common in the Western world are associated with a lack of fibre in the diet; these diseases are rare in communities which eat a high-fibre diet.

* Constipation. About 40 per cent of the British population think they are constipated and about 20 per cent take laxatives. The benefits of a diet higher in fibre, particularly insoluble fibre found in wholemeal bread, brown rice and wholegrain pasta, in treating constipation are now clear – and it's healthier and cheaper than taking laxatives.

* Diverticular disease. This is a disease of the large bowel which is characterised by small pouches in the wall of the bowel which can become inflamed. It's believed to be associated with a low-fibre diet, and increasing the fibre in the diet relieves the symptoms.

* Cancer of the large bowel. Development of this cancer is favoured by a low-fibre diet and there's good evidence that increasing the fibre in our diet may help to prevent it.

* Heart disease. A high level of cholesterol in the blood contributes to the furring-up of arteries which is the

foundation for heart attacks and strokes. A diet high in fibre, particularly soluble fibre which is found in fruit and vegetables as well as in oats and beans, helps to reduce the level of cholesterol in the blood and so reduce the risk of a heart attack.

* Diabetes is very uncommon in communities with diets high in fibre and increasing the fibre in our diet may reduce our risk of developing it.

* Gall-stones tend to form more easily when the diet is lacking in fibre.

* Other diseases where a low-fibre diet is implicated include:
    appendicitis
    haemorrhoids (piles)
    hiatus hernia
    varicose veins

FAT

Fat certainly helps to create fat! Incredible as it may seem, there are still diets on sale which advocate a high-fat (and low-carbohydrate) regime for losing weight. That's an unhealthy way of eating as well as an inefficient way of losing weight.

Fat really is the number one culprit in making so many of us overweight. On average, we get 40 per cent of our calories from fat. That seems impossible, but when you look at where the fat in our diet lurks, you can see that it is all too possible – even if you think you don't like fat and cut it off your meat. It's not just the fat you can see that counts, but also the furtive fat you can't see.

Cakes and biscuits, for example, which we think of as sweet things, in fact usually sock us with far more calories from the fat in them than from the sugar. Chocolate is a third fat and so is Cheddar cheese. Roast shoulder of lamb can be a quarter fat and even lean grilled rump steak still contains some fat.

Remember that, weight-for-weight, pure fat contains twice as many calories as pure protein or pure carbohydrates. But the big problem is not so much the 'pure' fat we can identify and so cut out – like the fat of butter and lard – but the fat bound up with other foods (such as with protein in cheese and with carbohydrate in cakes and pastries).

The BBC Diet is very effective at reducing the amount of fat you'll eat – which is why it's so effective in weight loss. All the diet plans are carefully formulated so you cut fat to the minimum; and the guidelines in chapter 9 (if you want to be more flexible) will really help you to cut the fat, too.

Reducing the amount of fat you eat is not only the surest way to lose weight: it's also going to help make you much healthier. Reducing fat, particularly animal fat, is going to help to reduce your risk of heart disease and even some types of cancer.

Protein and fat

Protein is an essential part of our diet, but it's virtually impossible for someone in the UK to go short of it – in fact we eat about twice as much protein as we need. The proportion of protein in our diet has remained about the same over this century, and the consensus of medical opinion is that we should keep the consumption at about the present level. With present-day medical knowledge, the high-protein diets recommended in the past make no nutritional sense. Weight-for-weight, protein contains more calories than carbohydrate.

The problem for those wanting to lose weight is that protein is very often bound up with fat. As we've seen, the protein in roast shoulder of lamb is bound up with 25 per cent fat and the protein in Cheddar cheese is bound up with

33 per cent fat. So what the dieter needs to do is find good sources of protein which aren't bound up with fat. Obviously some lean meat is all right and chicken and white fish are high in protein but low in fat. It's a myth, by the way, that only meat provides 'first class' protein – the protein of chicken and fish is just as nutritious. And by pairing beans, peas or lentils with rice or wholemeal bread or pasta, you end up with a complete protein meal – as well as providing only the tiniest traces of fat.

Where does the fat lurk?

It may be a bit of a surprise to see where, on average, we get our fat from in the food we eat. The guidelines for cutting down the fat in each of these categories are on pp. 99–104.

* **25 per cent of fat comes from meat and meat products.** This is not just fat we can see on things like chops, but the hidden fat in things like sausages, pies, pâtés and salami. Up to two-thirds of the calories in something like a meat pie may come from fat.

* **21 per cent of fat comes from butter and margarines.** Remember that even margarines labelled 'high in polyunsaturates' like sunflower margarine contain just as many calories as butter.

* **14 per cent of fat comes from cooking oils and fats.** It's possible, as *The BBC Diet* shows, to eliminate almost entirely this source of fat – and without too much pain!

* **11 per cent of fat comes from milk.** On average we drink quite a lot of milk, and, so, although whole milk only contains 4 per cent fat, the total amount of fat we consume from milk may be significant. Drinking half a pint – 10 fl oz (300 ml) – of milk a day is the equivalent of drinking a pint (600 ml) of single cream a week! That's why your note to the milkman says 'skimmed, please'!

* **7 per cent of fat comes from biscuits, cakes and pastries.** You don't need to stretch your imagination to know how to eliminate this source of fat when you want to lose weight!

* **7 per cent of fat comes from cream and cheese.** Cream is, of course, a no-no! Follow the guidelines for eating lower-fat cheeses.

* **15 per cent of fat comes from other foods.** Important things to watch for here are crisps or nuts which are high in fat and should be avoided while you're losing weight. The rest of this category is made up of fat from a wide variety of sources: if we've cut the fat in the other areas, we don't need to worry too much about this.

SUGAR

'Pure white and deadly' is how the nutritionist, Professor John Yudkin, has labelled refined sugar. It is the other significant factor for so many of us being above the weight we would like to be.

Just as with fat, you may think you don't eat a great deal of sugar. But on average we each consume nearly 2 lb (1 kg) of sugar a week in this country. A hundred years ago that's how much one person would eat in a whole year. Can you believe that you eat nearly a hundred pounds of the stuff a year? Well, if *you* don't, someone's making up the average by eating more!

But we all do eat more sugar than we could possibly imagine. Only half of the amount we eat is actually added by us to food – stirred into tea or coffee, sprinkled on cornflakes. The other half is added for us by food manufacturers. An average can of fizzy soft drink contains about 10 teaspoonfuls of sugar! That's as many calories, remember, as in 1¼ lb (550 g) of peas.

Sugar is all over the place: it's added to savoury sauces,

soups, baked beans, tinned vegetables and all manner of savoury things. It's even added to many breakfast cereals which try to promote a 'healthy' image.

You may now be beginning to see how we average 400–500 calories a day from sugar. Those are calories we can do without.

Sugar has what nutritionists call 'empty' calories – it has virtually no other nutrients at all. Sugar (and sugary products) are sometimes promoted as being 'high in energy' but that's just another way of saying 'high in calories'. It's a myth that we need sugar for energy – all food gives us energy! Energy is measured in calories and most of us are getting rather too much energy from our food as it is! We don't need 'instant energy' from sugar either: our bodies have already thought of that, and we have glucose in our bloodstream and glycogen (glucose and water) stored in our liver and muscles instantly available whenever we need them. We'd be dead if we didn't.

Remember that sugar is sugar is sugar. Glucose, fructose, maltose and dextrose are all sugar. Brown sugar is as fattening as white and is no better for you. And honey? That's virtually just sugar and water – refined by bees rather than machines!

You can now see why *The BBC Diet* is based on the following three principles:

* cutting down fat

* cutting down sugar

* increasing fibre.

With these three principles and the further one of starting to take exercise, this is the diet which has the latest scientific and medical facts behind it to back it up and help you lose weight!

6 Getting Yourself on Your Side

'Giving up smoking is easy; I've
done it many times.'

MARK TWAIN

Perhaps you feel like that about dieting: you've lost weight several times, haven't reached your target and have given up and put back on all the weight you've lost (and perhaps even added a little more).

The BBC Diet is very easy to follow and, as so many people have now proved, it is startlingly successful. Following it, you will lose weight, not feel hungry and still enjoy food. But that doesn't mean that it doesn't require some effort on your part, some willpower.

I'm not talking about some exceptional iron will, but I am talking about making a resolution that you want to lose weight, and being determined to do it. You've obviously already made one very significant commitment by buying and reading this book. Now this chapter is designed to help you build on that commitment and psych yourself up for achieving the weight loss that is your goal. There are a few very simple ways to prepare yourself and which will help you to succeed.

EVE'S TEMPTATION

And in this context it's just as likely to be Adam's! So many things that we want to do in life involve a little inner battle with ourselves. A personal example for me is writing. I *wanted* to write this book, of course – otherwise I wouldn't have agreed to do it. But as soon as I start writing, I can think of so many reasons to stop: 'it would be so nice to sit in the garden for a while' or 'it would be so good to read that book that's been sitting on my bookshelf for the past five years.' It's a strange part of human nature and it seems to be universal. St Paul, admittedly speaking on a more cosmic scale, wrote about 'the good things I want to do, I can't do and the bad things I don't want to do are the very things I do' – my paraphrase!

I am sure that you will recognise this phenomenon if you've tried to lose weight before. As soon as you go on a diet – even on one like *The BBC Diet*, when there's plenty to eat and you don't need to feel hungry – you get a sudden urge for a slice of Black Forest gâteau or chocolate fudge cake or double fish and chips! And the extraordinary thing is that it's usually a craving for something you haven't thought about for weeks anyway. The 'forbidden' suddenly has the most fatal allure. Well, let's leave the theological images of forbidden fruit, original sin and our fallen nature to one side – how do you deal with these feelings?

There's advice about coping with immediate temptation on p. 78 but this chapter is all about getting yourself into the frame of mind which can enable you to keep your eyes firmly fixed on your weight-loss goal – and not be distracted.

One advantage you do have over Eve, of course, is that you can reach for that apple!

WHY DO YOU WANT TO LOSE WEIGHT?

This may seem a rather superfluous question, but it's an important one. Spend a few minutes thinking of, and *writing down*, the reasons why you personally want to lose weight. Keeping this list by you will be one of your little shields in the battle against temptation. Your list might look something like this:

* 'I want to stand without any clothes on, look into a full-length mirror and smile.'

* 'I want to look down and see my feet again.'

* 'I want to buy myself a slinky red dress.'

* 'I want to get into a pair of 501s.'

* 'I want to look sexier.'

* 'I don't want to be breathless walking the dog.'

* 'I want to sunbathe on the beach this year.'

* 'I want to get slim for our silver wedding.'

* 'I want to get into the half of my wardrobe that I never wear.'

* 'I want to feel fitter.'

* 'I want to feel more self-confident.'

* 'I just want to feel right!'

Try to think of at least ten reasons of your own and write them down. Remember that the most powerful reasons are the ones you genuinely feel. Don't worry about how silly any of them may sound: you don't need to show them to anyone. Write down *your* reasons now.

ENLISTING HELP

Use your family and friends to help you to slim. If you're married, it's vital that you get your husband or wife to help you. Perhaps if your spouse is a little on the podgy side, you could slim together – that will certainly make it easier. If your spouse is unhelpful and says, 'I like you the way you are' then talk about some of the reasons you want to slim and explain, tactfully, that *you'd* feel much happier if you lost some weight.

Some people find it useful to slim with a friend – you can compare notes and support each other. You may or may not find it helpful to be competitive (hopefully your personalities will match in this respect) but on the whole it's probably better not to be, but rather to encourage and so reinforce each other's success.

You will also find it a good idea to let family and friends know not only that you are slimming, but also how much weight you're hoping to lose. Then you should give them progress reports. This may begin to bore them, but if at least they seem to be enthusiastic this will give you another boost. On the other hand, your personality may be such that you'd rather tell no one, slim in secret and wait for unsolicited comments. Again, do what suits you best.

KEEPING A FOOD DIARY

Let's talk a little more about the most immediately important factor determining our weight: how much we eat. If you know exactly what you eat, you'll know why you're fat. You might find it rather unnecessary for me to suggest that you should find out what you eat. 'I already know – only too well!' you may exclaim.

But, in fact, it's been shown many times that people don't really have a fully accurate picture of what they eat – unless they carefully write it down as they go along. We all forget

FOOD DIARY

When?	Where?	What?	With whom?
8.10 am	In the kitchen	Cup of tea with 2 teaspoons of sugar and ordinary milk. 2 slices white toast with butter and marmalade.	The children
10.40 am	In the office	1 coffee with two sugars and ordinary milk. 1 jam doughnut.	Ann and Sue
12.50 pm	In the canteen	Fried fish in batter, chips and peas. Ice-cream. Tea with two sugars and ordinary milk.	Sue and Liz
3.45 pm	In the office	1 tea with ordinary milk and 2 sugars. Cream cake.	Alone
6.30 pm	Living-room	1 cheese and tomato sandwich. 1 cup of tea with ordinary milk and two sugars.	Husband and children
9.50 pm	Living-room	1/2 pint lager. Scotch egg and packet of cheese and onion crisps.	Husband

What were you doing?	Were you hungry?	How did you feel?	Comment
Trying to give them breakfast.	No	Harassed	Didn't notice what I was eating.
Gossiping	Yes	Relaxed	Didn't really enjoy doughnut
Chatting	No	Okay	Had fish and chips because I didn't fancy anything else.
Carried on working.	No	Bored	Wish I hadn't had the cake — something to do!
Talking and watching TV	No	Okay	Didn't feel like cooking after preparing children's meal.
Watching TV	Yes	Tired	Didn't notice what I was eating — was enjoying film.

the odd bag of crisps or the few chips left over from the children's plates that we eat absentmindedly. Also, writing down a few things associated with the process of eating – like what else you were doing and how you were feeling at the time – may provide some very helpful clues to maximising your weight loss.

So keep a 'food diary' just before you start to diet. Ideally, you should try to keep it for a week, but even a couple of days will be useful: try to include at least one weekday and one weekend day. The previous pages give an example of how a 'food diary' might look. Draw one up for yourself and fill it in in the same way (or see p. 400 for a blank version which you can photocopy).

When you've done your own food diary, go through it, and look at the things it can teach you about what you eat – and why you're fat! Did this contain fat? Did that contain sugar? What could I have had instead?

How can you cut down on the fat?

In our example of a 'food diary' you could have:

* had a low-fat spread instead of butter.

* used skimmed milk instead of whole milk.

* had fresh fruit instead of the doughnut and cream cake.

* had poached or grilled fish instead of fried. If your canteen at work doesn't provide it, pester them. I'm sure they'll be surprised at its popularity if they advertise it as the 'Slimmer's Choice'.

* had a baked potato or boiled potatoes instead of chips.

* had a low-fat fruit yoghurt instead of the ice-cream.

* had a proper meal in the evening so you wouldn't have had high-fat Scotch egg and crisps later.

How can you cut down on the sugar?

In the example, you could have:

* not had sugar in coffee and tea, weaning yourself off it or using sweeteners instead.

* had reduced-sugar marmalade or had a wholegrain breakfast cereal and fruit instead.

* had fresh fruit instead of the doughnut and cream cake.

How can you increase the fibre?

You could have:

* had wholemeal bread instead of white.

* had baked potato or boiled potatoes in their skins in place of the chips.

* had a portion of pasta or rice in the evening instead of the Scotch egg and crisps.

Now you've examined the fat, sugar and fibre content of your 'food diary', it's time to look at your pattern of eating and why you eat what and when you do.

* Why did you eat sometimes when you weren't hungry? It's easy to cut calories by breaking these habits and only eating when you are hungry.

* How do you say no to jam doughnuts and cream cakes? Working out how to and thinking what you will have instead, will help when you're on your diet and you have to face the temptation.

* How often did you snack? Only eat at regular mealtimes and don't be tempted to nibble, pick and eat on the move. If you want to snack, snack on fruit and vegetables (see p. 79).

* How often did you eat when you were doing something else? Watching television, it's easy to pile in food without noticing it, let alone enjoying it. When you eat, concentrate only on that and don't do anything else.

* Did you eat when you were bored or unhappy? Eating for reasons other than hunger can be a big contributor to excess calories.

HAVING A TARGET

Giving yourself a target, something to aim for, is going to help you to reach it. Having considered what's in chapter 2, decide how much weight you want to lose.

Be realistic, and while bearing the charts on p. 30 in mind, aim at a weight you know that you personally will be happy at. You then write down your target to make a 'contract'.

Making a 'contract' with ourselves is something we do all the time – we often give ourselves a 'reward' for achieving something. For example, 'I'll clean the kitchen floor, then I'll have a cup of coffee' or 'I'll mow the lawn and then I'll put my feet up.'

It's useful, to help you to succeed in your weight-loss target, actually to write down a contract with yourself which builds in some small rewards for achieving targets along the way. Your contract might look something like the example at the top of the opposite page.

It's a good idea to pin this contract up where you will see it often – on the fridge door perhaps! It's also useful to pin up with it a full-length photograph of yourself as you are now. You can then use your imagination to think how you *will* be!

You may find it more helpful to sign a contract with someone else – like your husband or wife or a friend – and, if you're lucky, get him or her to agree to give you the rewards. This might look something like the contract at the bottom of the opposite page:

I, John Brown

promise myself that I shall lose 15 lb

After I have lost the first 5 lb I shall buy

myself a set of golf balls

After I have lost the next 5 lb I shall buy myself

a new pair of sunglasses

And after I have lost the whole 15 lb I shall buy

myself a new pair of golfing trousers

John Brown   3rd February

I, Sue Brown promise to lose 1½ stone

and I, John Brown promise to help her

After she has lost 7 lb, I shall give her

a bouquet of flowers

After she has lost the next 7 lb, I shall give her

three breakfasts in bed and after she has lost

the whole 1½ stone I shall give her

a weekend away to a surprise destination

Sue Brown   John Brown, 3rd February

COPING WITH TEMPTATION

Now you've two little shields to help you cope with those times you are tempted to stray off the straight and narrow:

* Your list of reasons for wanting to lose weight.

* Your contract with yourself or with someone else.

Keep them handy and look at them and think about them if any wicked thoughts connected with double cream or chocolate do float into your head.

How else do you cope with temptation?

Safe shopping

* If you live on your own, you need to make sure you don't buy tempting sugary or fatty food. If you live with your family, you may need to continue to buy such things for them – in which case, follow the strategies below.

* Always make a list before you go shopping and promise yourself you won't make impulse purchases.

* Don't shop on an empty stomach. If you're not hungry as you walk around supermarket shelves you'll be less prone to temptation.

* Start looking at food labels – sugar and fat are often hidden in the most unlikely foods.

* Beware of the chocolate at the checkout!

* If you know you always buy cream cakes at the bakers because they're so delicious, start buying your bread from the supermarket.

Food in the house

Work out some strategies if your family won't take too kindly to your not buying their favourite cakes and biscuits just because you're slimming!

* Make sure you buy plenty of non-fattening snack alternatives for yourself so that you can always turn away from the biscuits and chocolate. Fresh fruit is your great friend – make sure that you buy plenty of it. If you do feel hungry or are about to attack that box of chocolates, eat an apple or some other fresh fruit. If you're still tempted, eat another apple!

* If you do buy cakes or packets of crisps or chocolate for someone else, put them into separate bags and write 'Jane's' or 'Gary's' on it. Then if you think of eating it, remember you're stealing!

* Have in the fridge ready-prepared sticks of carrot, celery, peppers, radishes, cucumber, courgettes etc. Keep them crisp in a bowl of water or a polythene bag and eat them if you fancy something savoury.

* Look again at your food diary (pp. 72–3). Think of any problem areas you have and work out in advance ways of dealing with them.

The principles in this book don't just apply to slimmers – eating less fat and sugar and more fibre is healthier for everyone. So when you start slimming you can begin to change your whole family's diet to a more healthy one. This would also benefit you because you don't have to cook separate meals. The secret with changing a family's eating habits is to take it slowly. Don't cut out too many of their favourite foods all at once. For example, you could give them a healthy and low-fat main course, and apple pie and custard or whatever they want, as a pudding. Meanwhile, you'll be having fresh fruit. When they insist on chips, you can have a baked potato, brown rice or pasta.

I know some dieters prefer to cook and eat separately from the rest of the family, but it's far easier to stick to a diet if you're eating at least some of the same food. It does make sense too, to think of their health as well as your figure.

WATCHING YOUR PROGRESS

It's a good idea to write down your progress – it will help to encourage you. So, following the example below (or see the blank version on pages 403 and 404), write down your weight every week. Write the date alongside.

Date	Weight

Keeping this record should be a very pleasant task!

Try to weigh yourself at the same time of day each week, in the same state of dress (or preferably, undress) and on the same pair of scales. Remember that weight can fluctuate on a day-to-day basis because of water loss or retention so, in fact, a weekly weigh-in is going to give you a much more accurate reflection of your real progress than a daily one possibly can.

Now, for your measurements!

Date	Bust/chest	Waist	Hips	Thighs	Upper arm

You may find it helpful to keep a note like this of your measurements as well as your weight (see the blank version on pages 405 and 406). Do this every couple of weeks. You may find it easier to ask someone else to take the measurements for you. Remember to take the measurements in the same way and at the same points each time.

KNOWING YOURSELF

It's important to assess realistically the kind of person you are, so that you can get your personality on your side and work with it and not against it.

* Do you like following a diet absolutely strictly? If so, you can follow one of the diet plans to the letter.

* Do you prefer a diet plan which is more flexible? If so, you can still follow *The BBC Diet* by following the guidelines in chapter 9. Alternatively follow one of the plans and use your knowledge from the guidelines to vary it when you want to.

* Can you be 'moderate'? Are you the kind of person who can have just one chocolate and then continue on your diet for the rest of the week? Or, if you have one chocolate, do you think 'oh, I've now broken my diet' and have another and another and another to drown your sorrows! One chocolate isn't going to affect your rate of weight loss, but a boxful will. So if you're in the second category of personality here, don't be tempted by even one chocolate.

* Do you have to have a quick result or are you more patient? Would you prefer to diet for a couple of weeks, then just eat sensibly for another few weeks, then diet again until you get down to your target weight? Or, would you prefer to slog on for a few weeks and keep going until you've reached your ideal weight? Either way of reaching your goal will work, but beware of going 'off' your diet, planning to go back 'on' in the near future, and then promptly forgetting all about it.

* Would you prefer to be able to cheat a little? Or do you want to be absolutely hard on yourself? Cheating a little is fine if you accept your weight loss will be a little slower than it would be otherwise. If you do cheat, be careful to avoid two traps: pretending you're not cheating and wondering why your weight loss isn't as quick as you had hoped; or getting into a spiral of deviating more and more from your diet so that you eventually pack it in altogether.

7 How to Follow
The BBC Diet

The three principles of *The BBC Diet* – less fat, less sugar, more fibre – are worked out for you here in eight different two-week diet plans. They are designed to be as flexible as possible so, although the plans are set out over a two-week period, you can choose to eat the meals in any order if you prefer. You can also interchange equivalent meals between days, for example, swopping one snack meal for another. Although a variety of food is important for a nutritious diet, you're not obliged to have as much variety as the plans suggest! You could, for example, eat the same thing for breakfast every day if you wanted to and you could eat the same thing for lunch a couple of days in the week.

There are also two ways of making *The BBC Diet* even more flexible and that's either by following one of the Flexible Plans in chapter 18 or by following the series of guidelines set out in chapter 9 – The DIY BBC Diet. This perhaps requires a little more thought to begin with, though the great advantage of it is that, once you've mastered the guidelines, you'll be totally in charge of how you follow the diet and you can be sure you'll make the right choices in the supermarket, or when eating out.

In practice, most people will probably use a mixture of two methods. Some people will prefer to follow a set plan but will find the guidelines useful when they need greater flexibility and others will follow the guidelines but use parts of the set plans now and again to give them ideas and to make sure they're on the right lines.

Another way of using the plans is to alternate them: you could have two weeks on The Quickfire Plan, followed by two weeks on The Middle Way, followed by two weeks on The Hearty-eating Plan. Or you could alternate between a couple of them. Alternating may actually be more effective for you as you may find it easier to continue to diet, after the quick initial weight loss, by having 'easier' and slightly 'harder' fortnights.

As all these plans are based on healthy, as well as slimming, eating, it's quite safe to continue on one **until you have reached your ideal weight** (see p. 30).

FOLLOWING THE SET PLANS

You'll find that each plan comes with its own daily and weekly allowances for skimmed milk (enough for breakfast and teas and coffees), low-fat spread and, in some plans, alcoholic drinks. Note these allowances carefully and do follow them – they're an important part of each plan. There is no restriction on coffee or tea but don't add any sugar to them and keep within your milk allowance. If you need to, use artificial sweeteners.

Don't drink any sweetened drinks. You can drink unlimited quantities of water, both still and sparkling, and no-cal drinks. You could also try low-cal commercial drinks or drink unsweetened natural fruit juice (but not more than 7 fl oz/200 ml a day). It is important, in fact, to drink plenty of water – this is not only needed when you increase your fibre intake but it will also help to fill you up. It's a good idea always to have a glass of mineral water or plain tap water with each meal.

Try not to skip breakfast. If you eat then, it really will help you from being tempted to snack later. Of course, this isn't a rigid rule; you could eat what you should eat for breakfast as a snack later in the day.

In some of the plans there is a weekly alcohol allowance

– but you're not obliged to drink it. If you want to lose weight quickly it's best to avoid alcohol. If you do want to drink alcohol, don't cut down on the food you're eating. Remember that alcohol only contains calories and no nutrients. So if you do drink, remember that you're adding calories and are slowing down your weight loss.

Where quantities or weights of food are given, then you should obviously follow them. Where no quantities are given, then you are free to eat as much as you like of that particular food. Some people find this a little too liberal and wonder if they aren't accidentally going to be eating too many calories. I assure you that you needn't worry. For example, in some recipes, I've said something like 4–6 oz (100–175 g) mushrooms. This is a suggested quantity for a reasonable amount. The difference in calorie content between 4 and 6 oz of mushrooms is in fact infinitesimal – there are only about 100 calories in 2 lb (1 kg) mushrooms! Similarly, there are only 100 calories in 1½ lb (750 g) peppers, which is why items like this – and lettuce, cucumber and tomato – can be eaten freely. If you *were* (by some extraordinary means!) able to eat 100 calories' worth of items like these, then you certainly wouldn't have room for much else! In such cases the sheer bulk of the food is the limiting factor to the number of calories you can take in. But do beware: this only applies to certain foods which I've listed. With other food, you may be able to pack in too many calories and so the quantity of those *is* given. Always keep in mind those comparisons: about 1 oz (25 g) butter having more calories than 10 oz (275 g) potatoes and 1 lb (450 g) chocolates having more calories than 10 lb (4.5 kg) of apples and then you'll understand why some foods are on the 'free' list and some are strictly controlled – and yet others are not eaten at all for the duration of your diet.

NOTES ON TECHNIQUES AND RECIPES

'Dry-frying'

This technique is fundamental to reducing the amount of fat in your diet. Many foods are quite low in calories in themselves and only become fattening when we start adding fat to them. But it is possible to 'fry' without adding any fat at all. Here's how.

You need a thick-bottomed, heavy, non-stick frying-pan. This is essential. You need to use less heat than you normally would when you fry something; so it will take longer and requires a little more patience. If you're frying chopped onions, for example, put them in the pan over a medium heat and stir them constantly with a wooden spoon until they soften. Be patient, keep stirring, and you will find that they start to brown. It's difficult to get them *as* brown as when you add oil. If they begin to stick, add just 1 tablespoon of water and stir well where they are sticking; turn the heat down a little lower and carry on stirring. A little water will always help things to 'unstick' but you don't want to add too much or things will start simmering in water and then you won't get a 'fried' taste but rather a 'boiled' one. By the way, the reason for this is simple: if onions cook *in* water, their temperature cannot go above the boiling temperature of water –100°C. The whole point about *frying* is to get food to a higher temperature as changes then occur which favourably affect the taste. In the case of onions, the natural sugars in them caramelise and so the onions go brown. By using the technique of 'dry-frying', you can get onions to such a temperature that they do begin to go brown and have that lovely taste – provided you're careful and patient.

This technique can be used for anything you would normally shallow fry in fat – garlic, mushrooms, peppers, meat and fish. Meat will be sealed and go brown. It may stick a little, but you can add water or wine or stock to stir into the residue, scrape it up, and ensure all the flavour is in your sauce (see individual recipes for further examples of this technique). The only thing I would say is that while fish like mackerel and trout can be 'dry-fried' fairly easily if you're careful, fragile white fish is better if grilled – it tends to break up when you try to fry it.

Frying-pans and woks

A wok is very useful for stir-frying a large amount of food in a very small amount of oil. However, in my experience it's not good for 'dry-frying' as the food tends to stick. So, when you're adding no oil at all – as I recommend while you're losing weight – use a non-stick, thick-based frying-pan rather than a wok (unless you happen to have a non-stick wok).

If you're cooking a stir-fry recipe for three or four people, say, you could use a wok and use about a tablespoon of oil, which is about 120 calories. This isn't much divided by three or four, but the reason I suggest *not* using oil if you're cooking just for yourself is that 120 would be probably *more* calories than you're getting from the vegetables, chicken, pork or whatever you're frying. So try to 'dry-fry' for yourself; only stir-fry for more than two people using a tablespoon of oil.

Using oil to coat foil or a baking tray

For this cooking technique you use a piece of kitchen paper and pour a little oil onto it. Then grease your foil or baking tray with it very thinly and wipe off any excess with some more paper. In this way, you should be able to grease foil or a baking tray using less than half a teaspoon of oil – which is important when oil is 40 calories a teaspoonful!

Parmesan cheese

In several recipes, I recommend using freshly grated Parmesan. Parmesan is a medium-fat cheese, but I'm suggesting using it in very small quantities at a time. Its great advantage is that it is highly flavoured and so a small amount of it makes its mark. I don't really think it's worth buying ready grated Parmesan – it looks like sawdust and doesn't taste much better! If you want to use something else, use finely grated, half-fat Cheddar-type cheese.

Chicken stock

Several recipes call for chicken stock and I do suggest that you make your own and freeze it (see p. 348). If you haven't done it before, you'll find that it is easier than you think. You can, however, use stock made from a cube if you want to. If you're a vegetarian, you could use a vegetarian stock cube, water that you've used to cook vegetables in, or even just water.

Melba wholemeal toast and crispy pitta bread

One of the great advantages of making toast or preparing pitta bread in the following way is that you seem to get twice the quantity for the same number of calories.

Melba toast is very easy to make.

Lightly toast some wholemeal bread in the normal way. Now cut off the crusts and slice horizontally through the bread so that you are left with two slices, each toasted on one side and soft and untoasted on the inner half. Pull off from the untoasted side any soft bits of bread. This helps to make it crispy and has the happy side-effect of reducing the calories!

Now put the toast in a warm oven for a few minutes until the bread is crisp and browning on the previously untoasted side. Or place the toast, untoasted side up, under a grill and heat until it's crisp and browning.

Melba toast is delicious with things like Tapénade (p. 237), Carrot and dill pâté (p. 237) and Hummus (p. 238). It's so delicious that you don't need any added fat spread on it and, of course, you do get two slices for every one slice of wholemeal bread.

Wholemeal pitta bread can be dealt with in a similar way. Heat the pitta bread in a moderate oven (gas mark 4, 350°F, 180°C), cut it in half and then slice it through horizontally (it naturally comes apart horizontally to make a pouch when you cut it in two). Pull off any soft pieces from the inside, and warm through again in the oven until it is crisp. By the way, if you've got a freezer you can store pitta bread easily and use it one piece at a time.

Alcohol

Several recipes suggest adding alcohol (although there's always an alternative if you don't want to). You may be surprised at this as it seems to be adding calories recklessly. The calories in an alcoholic drink come from two ingredients: sugar and from the pure alcohol itself (see p. 107). As I'm mostly suggesting the addition of just a few tablespoons of alcohol the calories are fairly insignificant. Furthermore, in the heating process, the alcohol evaporates, making the calories more insignificant still. In the few recipes where I suggest using more than a tablespoon or so of alcohol, I suggest using *dry* wine so there are virtually no calories from any sugar content.

Eggs

Eggs are an excellent food in moderation (3–4 a week) as they are a good source of protein and an average egg contains only 80 calories.

The Department of Health guidelines on 'safe' egg-eating

are still in force at the time of writing. These are that no one should eat raw eggs and that the very young, the old, pregnant women, and those at special risk (for example whose immune system is suppressed by illness or medication) should not eat lightly cooked eggs, but only eggs which are cooked until solid.

There is one recipe in this book (*The BBC Diet* chocolate mousse p. 329) which does contain raw eggs and there are some where the eggs are lightly cooked, so you should use your own discretion in these cases.

Yoghurt and fromage frais

These feature quite often in the recipes as 'creamy' ingredients.

* **Low-fat natural yoghurt.** This has an insignificant fat content and is very low in calories – so low that you can use it freely. It's good with fruit and for puddings and mousses and for salad dressings, but it's not so good for cooking as it separates when heated. It is possible to stabilise it by mixing into it a little cornflour stirred into a little skimmed milk: you then can bring it to the boil. But in most dishes, it's best to stir in the yoghurt off the heat when you've finished cooking everything else.

* **Greek yoghurt.** This is a much creamier and thicker yoghurt because it has been strained. It tastes delicious, but unfortunately it is higher in fat. There are two kinds: sheep's milk yoghurt which is about 8 per cent fat and cow's milk which is about 10 per cent. (Remember that 'ordinary' milk is about 4 per cent fat while single cream is 18 per cent: double cream is 48 per cent!) If you want to eat large quantities of yoghurt, use low-fat natural yoghurt instead. If you're only using 1 or 2 tablespoons, Greek yoghurt is fine.

    Greek yoghurt is more stable than low-fat natural

yoghurt when you heat it but it is still best to take the dish off the heat before adding it.

* Fromage frais. The name suggests that this is a cheese, though in fact it's a lovely thick creamy substance which doesn't taste of cheese at all. It is suitable for use in savoury and sweet dishes – but again, it isn't stable when boiled, so if you're adding it to a hot dish, add at the end and off the heat.

Fromage frais comes in two kinds: the very low-fat version which is less than 1 per cent fat and the version which is 8 per cent. The 1 per cent version is dryer and grainier, while the 8 per cent, of course, is creamier. Only use the 8 per cent version in 1 or 2 tablespoon quantities at a time; if you want to use more than that, use the very low-fat version.

You can now buy small pots of fruit-flavoured fromage frais. However, if you're going to have one of these, check that it's a diet version – even if it says 'low-fat' it may have added sugar. (This also, of course, applies to any fruit yoghurt.)

I should just add that I've heard some people get confused between fromage frais and crème fraîche. The French language is the only thing they have in common. Crème fraîche is a yummy, naturally soured fresh cream – but sadly it contains about 35 per cent fat. So it's out!

By the way, some pots of fromage frais give a percentage of fat content in French (*matière grasse*). The version which says 8 per cent in English may for example say 40 per cent in French. This is accounted for by the fact that the English percentage is a proportion of the total weight of the product *including* water; the French percentage is the proportion of fat 'in dry matter' – in other words *excluding* the water content. Any percentage of fat that I quote in this book uses the English system.

I mention this because someone wrote to me after the first *BBC Diet* book was published telling me that I was wrong in saying that Brie had a lower fat content than Cheddar. He'd seen a French label which said that Brie was 60 or 70 per cent fat. But that doesn't mean that if you eat 100 g of Brie that you take in 60 or 70 g of fat! If you take the water into account (Brie contains more and is therefore softer than Cheddar) then, weight-for-weight, Brie will give you less fat than Cheddar – about 23 g per 100 g as opposed to Cheddar's 34 g per 100 g.

Sorry if this is confusing – understanding it isn't obligatory if you want to lose weight! All you need to do is follow the guidelines or one of the set plans.

8 Which Diet Plan to Choose

The Quickfire Plan	} 1000 calories
The Short, Sharp Shock	
The Middle Way	
The Easy Way	
The Vegetarian Plan	} 1250 calories
The Gourmet Plan	
The No-bother Plan	
The Slower But Sure Plan	} 1500 calories
The Hearty-eating Plan	

This is a summary of what each plan is all about, so that you can choose the best one for you. There is some advice about who should follow which plan, but you can follow any which takes your fancy. Also, you can alternate weeks or fortnights on different plans: I haven't worked out (meaning I *can't* work out!) the number of possible permutations, but I defy you to get bored!

If you don't want to follow a set plan, look at the next chapter *The DIY BBC Diet* which contains a series of guidelines rather than suggested menus.

THE QUICKFIRE PLAN

set plan p. 108 ✱ *flexible plan p. 180*

The Quickfire Plan provides the lowest number of calories you should go down to for safe and yet quick and effective weight loss. Anyone can use this plan for rapid results but all men and women of average height and who are quite active, will achieve satisfactory weight loss on the other plans. This one is mainly for women of below average height or who are very inactive. However, once you're losing weight steadily, you could try alternating with one of the other plans.

Look through the recipes to decide whether you prefer this plan to the Short, Sharp Shock. They have the same calorie counts, but this plan is based on more modern, slightly 'fancier' food than the Short, Sharp Shock.

THE SHORT, SHARP SHOCK

set plan p. 117

The Short, Sharp Shock provides the lowest number of calories you should go down to for safe and yet quick and effective weight loss. Anyone can use this plan for rapid results but all men and women of average height and who are quite active, will achieve satisfactory weight loss on the other plans. This one is mainly for women of below average height or who are very inactive. However, once you're losing weight steadily, you could try alternating with one of the other plans.

Look through the recipes to decide whether you prefer this plan to the Quickfire Plan. They have the same calorie counts, but this plan is based on more traditional, slightly plainer food than the Quickfire.

THE MIDDLE WAY

set plan p. 126

This plan is designed so that most women (unless they're of very small build or very inactive) will lose weight at a very satisfactory rate. All men will quickly lose weight on it.

Look through the recipes to decide whether you prefer this plan to the Easy Way. They have the same calorie counts, but this plan is based on more traditional, slightly plainer food than the Easy Way.

THE EASY WAY

set plan p. 135

This plan is designed so that most women (unless they're of very small build or very inactive) will lose weight at a very satisfactory rate. All men will quickly lose weight on it.

Look through the recipes to decide whether you prefer this plan to the Middle Way. They have the same calorie counts, but this plan is based on more modern, slightly 'fancier' food than the Middle Way.

THE VEGETARIAN PLAN

set plan p. 144 * flexible plan p. 190

This plan is designed so that most women (unless they're of very small build or very inactive) will lose weight at a very satisfactory rate. All men will quickly lose weight on it.

It's designed to appeal to all vegetarians and others who feel like having a change from meat- or fish-based dishes.

THE GOURMET PLAN

set plan p. 153 ✱ *flexible plan p. 199*

This plan is designed so that most women (unless they're of very small build or very inactive) will lose weight at a very satisfactory rate. All men will quickly lose weight on it.

It's for those who love their food and want to eat really tempting meals while they lose weight.

THE NO-BOTHER PLAN

flexible plan p. 219

This is a 'middle-way' flexible plan using convenience foods or very easy to prepare 'no-recipe' meals. It's satisfactory for most women unless they're of below average height or very inactive. If you are such a woman you could use this plan and increase your physical activity. Nearly all men will lose weight quickly on this plan.

THE SLOWER BUT SURE PLAN

set plan p. 162

Most men find that they lose weight at a very satisfactory rate with this plan and this will also be the case for most women who also increase their physical activity (see chapter 21).

Look through the recipes to decide whether you prefer this plan to the Hearty-eating Plan. They have the same calorie counts, but this plan is based on more traditional, slightly plainer food than the Hearty-eating Plan.

THE HEARTY-EATING PLAN

set plan p. 171 ✱ *flexible plan p. 210*

Most men find that they lose weight at a very satisfactory rate with this plan and this will also be the case for most women who also increase their physical activity (see chapter 21).

Look through the recipes to decide whether you prefer this plan to the Slower But Sure Plan. They have the same calorie counts, but this plan is based on more modern, slightly 'fancier' food than the Slower But Sure.

9 The DIY BBC Diet

To follow *The BBC Diet* you can choose one of the eight set plans which come later in this book or pick one of the five flexible plans, *or* use the guidelines in this chapter to create your own completely flexible plan to suit your lifestyle.

This last option might sound a bit more hit and miss than a conventional diet which lays down exactly what you may and may not eat but, if you do follow the guidelines carefully, you will cut down your calories sufficiently and lose weight effectively. Remember that it's important to follow the 'increasing your fibre' guidelines as well as those for 'decreasing the fat and sugar'. Increasing your fibre will make it easy for you to cut down on the fat and sugar without feeling hungry.

The advantage of this flexible plan is that *you* are in control. In any situation – in the supermarket, in a restaurant, cooking for yourself or family or friends – you'll always know how to choose the slimming options. You won't need to refer to a plan continually and you'll have fixed within your mind the knowledge which will enable you to stay slim and healthy.

A modified – and more liberal! – version of these guidelines is to be found in chapter 24 for when you're down to your ideal weight and want to keep it that way.

Remember, *The BBC Diet* is based on three principles:

* cutting down fat

* cutting down sugar

* increasing fibre.

WHERE'S THE FAT?

In chapter 5, we saw the percentages of where most of the fat comes from in the average British diet. Here they are again to remind you:

* 25 per cent from meat and meat products

* 21 per cent from butter and margarine

* 14 per cent from cooking oils and fats

* 11 per cent from milk

* 7 per cent from biscuits, cakes and pastries

* 7 per cent from cheese and cream

* 15 per cent from other foods

Here's how to cut that fat down.

Cutting down the fat from meat and meat products

* Meat products like pies, pasties, sausages, pâtés and salami can be very high in fat. As already mentioned, half the calories in a sausage and nearly two-thirds of the calories in a meat pie may be fat. Don't eat these products while you're trying to lose weight.

* Choose white chicken or turkey meat and remove the skin. Your portion size should be 3–4 oz (75–100 g). Remember that duck and goose are quite fatty.

* Choose lean cuts of meat and trim off visible fat. Your portion size should be 2–3 oz (50–75 g).

* Choose white fish as it is low in fat. Your portion size can be 4–5 oz (100–150 g). Even fatty fish like herring and mackerel is not too high in calories. Choose tinned fish, like tuna and sardines, packed in brine or water rather than oil.

* Always grill meat or fish rather than fry – this reduces the fat content of food very significantly. Alternatively, 'dry-fry' (see p. 86), microwave, steam or poach in water or skimmed milk.

* When cooking mince, choose the leanest you can buy. Your portion size should be 2–3 oz (50–75 g). Pour off all the fat after 'dry-frying' (see p. 86), or cover with water, bring slowly to the boil, simmer gently for a couple of minutes, pour off the now fatty water and then proceed with your recipe.

* In casseroles and other similar dishes cut down the amount of meat you would normally use. Remember even lean red meat has a significant fat content. To supplement the meat, add pulses like beans, lentils, split peas or chick peas.

Cutting down the fat from butter and margarine

* Switch to a low-fat spread such as Gold or Outline. Limit your intake of low-fat spread to ½ oz (15 g) a day (about 2 teaspoonfuls). Spread very thinly, this is enough for four slices of bread (wholemeal, of course) or two slices and a baked potato. (I know you don't measure low-fat spread normally in teaspoonfuls: if you scrape your knife tip very gently once across the packet, you'll end up with about ¼ oz or 10 g.) Remember, ½ oz (15 g) of low-fat

spread has about 50 calories, ½ oz (15 g) of butter or margarine has about 100.

* Try making sandwiches with the low-fat spread on one slice of bread rather than on both; if the filling is moist, try not adding any spread at all.

Cutting down the fat from cooking oils and fats

* Do not use cooking oils and fats while you're losing weight. Remember, 1 tablespoon of oil contains 120 calories. Grill, poach, steam or microwave instead.

* Use the technique of 'dry-frying' (see p. 86).

* Don't eat anything which you know has lard, cooking fat or oil added to it. That includes many ready-made dishes, bottled mayonnaise and salad creams (read the labels). Remember mayonnaise is largely oil and therefore packed with calories. Use low-fat natural yoghurt, thinned with a little wine vinegar, as a delicious alternative to both mayonnaise and vinaigrette or French dressing.

* When you're making chips for the family (and very occasionally for yourself when you've got to your ideal weight!) you can cut down the fat considerably. Cut your chips thickly (so that weight-for-weight there's a lower surface area to absorb the fat) and then fry them quickly in hot oil (hot oil seeps into the chips less than cooler oil). Again use an oil high in polyunsaturates and don't re-use it (which causes it to become saturated fat). Finally, shake off as much oil as possible and then, before serving, drain the chips on kitchen paper to get rid of any remaining fat.

* For your health's sake and that of your family, use polyunsaturated oil rather than hard cooking fats or oils just labelled 'cooking oil'. Find a 'named' oil like

sunflower, safflower or groundnut as these, particularly the first two, are high in polyunsaturates. Olive oil, which is also healthy (high in monounsaturates) is strongly flavoured and can therefore make its mark in a dish in very small quantities.

Cutting down the fat from milk

* Use only skimmed milk when you're losing weight. You can have up to 10 fl oz (300 ml) a day. Skimmed milk contains virtually no fat at all but still has all the protein and calcium of ordinary milk (indeed, a slightly higher percentage of each).

Cutting down the fat from biscuits, cakes and pastries

* While you're losing weight don't eat any of these products which are basically just sweetened fat. Fresh fruit is your slimming alternative.

Cutting down the fat from cream and cheese

* Here are those percentages again: double cream is 48 per cent fat! Whipping cream is 35 per cent fat and even single cream is 18 per cent fat! All cream is OUT if you want to lose weight.

* Use low-fat substitutes for cream such as low-fat natural yoghurt which is virtually fat-free. You can eat as much natural low-fat yoghurt and 1 per cent fromage frais as you like or 1–2 tablespoons of either 8 per cent fromage frais or Greek yoghurt per day (see p. 90).

* Cheddar cheese is about 33 per cent fat, Stilton about 40 per cent fat, and cream cheese about 50 per cent fat. As they contain more water, soft cheeses tend to contain less fat: Camembert, Brie and Edam are all about 23 per cent

fat. One of these last three should be your choice and you can eat about 1oz (25 g) a day.

✱ Cottage cheese is only about 4 per cent fat so if you like it, you're really onto a winner. You can eat it freely. I'm told (by Delia Smith, no less) that it's good stirred into mashed potatoes. That sounds fine if you don't add any other fat – you could always also add some skimmed milk.

✱ Try the new half-fat Cheddar-type cheeses which are about 14 per cent fat. Some of them are rather bland but they seem to be improving all the time. You can have up to 1½ oz (40 g) of this type of cheese.

✱ When using cheese in cooking, you could use less of a stronger flavoured variety – and perhaps add a little mustard to enhance the flavour.

Cutting down the rest of the fat in your diet

✱ Cut out all salted snacks – crisps, nuts and all those other strangely-shaped objects which are nothing but salted fat. Even so-called low-fat crisps are out, as even they still deliver nearly half their calories from fat.

✱ Eggs have sometimes had a bad press, but on the whole they're not a very significant contribution to the fat in our diet. It's true that egg yolks are high in cholesterol but, provided you're not eating a dozen or more eggs a week, the amount of cholesterol they produce is fairly insignificant. Three or four eggs a week should be your maximum. Use them instead of meat or fish for a main meal. A two-egg omelette with a non-fatty filling made with no added fat in a non-stick pan is a tasty low-calorie meal. A fresh herb omelette with a yoghurt and tarragon-vinegar dressed salad is a banquet!

* Most fruit and vegetables contain only minimal quantities of fat (until we try to improve on nature). One that contains a significant quantity is avocado. Don't eat them when you're losing weight.

WHERE'S THE SUGAR?

Remember that, on average, we each eat about a hundredweight of sugar a year: getting on for 2 lb (just under a kilo) a week. That's how sugar is giving us a staggering 400–500 calories a day. Remember also that when cutting down on sugar, we're only cutting down on calories: we get virtually no other nutrients from sugar at all.

* Don't take sugar in tea or coffee. Even if you have a sweet tooth, you really can learn to enjoy them without sugar. This is a simple change to make to reduce your sugar consumption for life.

* You need to make up your own mind about swapping sugar for artificial sweeteners. If you have a craving for sweet things you need to master it so you only indulge occasionally. I don't think artificial sweeteners help you to do this. By the way, there is one artificial sweetener, Sorbitol, used in most diabetic sweets and chocolates, which contains as many calories as sugar. So, if you use them, make sure you are using sweeteners designed for slimmers.

* Cut out fizzy canned drinks which are high in sugar. Either switch to low-cal or no-cal drinks or, better, drink sparkling mineral water with ice and lemon, or unsweetened fruit juices.

* Cut out sweet snacks, biscuits, chocolates, cakes or keep them for *very* occasional treats – choose fresh fruit instead where, remember, the sugar is well wrapped up in lots of fibre.

* Use tinned fruit packed in natural fruit juice rather than sugar syrup.

* Don't add sugar to your breakfast cereal and first check on the label to see if the manufacturer hasn't been there before you!

* Read the labels before you consume anything from a packet or can and avoid those which have added sugar.

* If you are buying processed food look for labels proclaiming 'reduced-sugar' or 'no added sugar'. So many things now – from baked beans to jams – offer a 'reduced-sugar' choice.

* Even reduced-sugar jams contain significant calories, so go sparingly with them.

* When you're making cakes, pies and other sweet things for the family (and very occasionally for yourself!) gradually try to cut down the amount of sugar you add. Aim over a few weeks to cut it by half. If there are complaints (though with most things there probably won't be) increase the sugar a little next time. You should be able to get approval and still reduce the sugar content of your family's diet!

WHERE'S THE FIBRE?

Fibre-rich foods include:

wholemeal bread
wholemeal flour
brown rice
wholemeal pasta
wholemeal breakfast cereals
porridge oats
bulgar (or burghul) wheat
other grains (e.g. millet and buckwheat)

lentils
peas (from split to frozen)
beans (of all kinds from baked to cannellini)
chick peas
sweetcorn
potatoes (baked or boiled in the skin)
green leafy vegetables (e.g. spinach)
dried fruits

* Try to start the day with muesli or a wholemeal breakfast cereal with no added sugar.

* Eat 2–4 slices of wholemeal bread a day. Remember that bread helps to fill you without fattening you. If you need to spread it with something, use a thin smear of low-fat spread from your allowance. Make sure you get 'wholemeal', which contains more fibre, rather than just 'brown' or 'wheatmeal'. White bread isn't 'bad', it's just that it contains only a quarter of the fibre of wholemeal.

* With your main meal try to have a helping of one of the following:
    potatoes (up to 8 oz, 225 g), scrubbed not peeled, either baked or boiled
    brown rice (up to 3 oz, 75 g, dry weight)
    wholewheat pasta (up to 3 oz, 75 g, dry weight)
    bulgar wheat (up to 3 oz, 75 g, dry weight)

* Try to eat a portion of peas or beans or other pulses once a day.

* Eat at least one other portion of fresh vegetables a day. All vegetables contain some fibre, but the really fibre-rich ones are those listed above. Salad vegetables like lettuce, tomatoes, cucumbers and celery don't contain very much fibre, but you can eat them freely as they also don't contain many calories.

* Eat two or three pieces of fresh fruit every day. Again, all fruit contains some fibre, though it's not particularly rich in it. It will help to fill you up, though, without providing too many calories.

* Dried fruit is higher in fibre but is also higher in calories so don't nibble too much 'neat'. Once you've soaked and cooked it, it contains much more water, so, weight-for-weight, contains fewer calories.

WHERE ELSE CAN WE CUT CALORIES?

In one word: alcohol. The average person takes perhaps 10 per cent of their daily calorie consumption from alcohol. This is drinking perhaps two or three drinks a day. You can cut these 200–300 calories at a stroke. Whether you want to or not is another matter. You may decide you'd rather lose weight a little more slowly and continue to drink moderately. It's important to remember that alcohol is 'empty' calories – supplying us with no nutrients. So don't substitute alcohol for food; if you want to lose weight on 1000 calories a day, you must add your calories from alcohol to this and accept that your weight loss will be slightly less rapid.

Very roughly – and as accurately as any of us needs to know – one glass of wine and half a pint of beer and one single (pub measure) of spirits with a mixer are about 100 calories each. You should stick to only one measure of one of them a day if you want to lose weight. Each of those measures contains one unit of alcohol. For your health's sake:

* men should not drink more than 21 units of alcohol a week – that's three a day.

* women should not drink more than 14 units of alcohol a week – that's two a day.

Safeguarding your health will also safeguard your figure.

10 The Quickfire Plan

(1000 calories a day)

The Quickfire Plan provides the lowest number of calories you should go down to for safe and yet quick and effective weight loss. Anyone can use this plan for rapid results but all men and women of average height and who are quite active, will achieve satisfactory weight loss on the other plans. This one is mainly for women of below average height or who are very inactive. However, once you're losing weight steadily, you could try alternating with one of the other plans.

Look through the recipes to decide whether you prefer this plan to the Short, Sharp Shock (see p. 117). They have the same calorie counts, but this plan is based on more modern, slightly 'fancier' food than the Short, Sharp Shock.

Remember the plan is completely flexible. The set plan isn't a magic formula. There's no need to eat chicken on Tuesday or tuna on Thursday if you don't feel like it, or if it's inconvenient. You can interchange any of the meals for an equivalent one. Remember, though, that variety of food is important for a nutritious diet.

You can have your snack meal in the evening instead of at lunchtime if it is easier. Remember, too, that you don't have to eat everything that's on the plan if you're feeling full!

There's a flexible version of this diet plan on p. 180, where you will find a lot more choice for breakfasts, snack meals and main meals.

These are the additional allowances for the Quickfire Plan (these are sometimes mentioned in the plans but, of course, you may use them as and when you like):

Daily allowance   10 fl oz (300 ml) skimmed milk
Weekly allowance   3 oz (75 g) low-fat spread

Other drinks:
Unlimited tap, still or carbonated water
Unlimited no-cal drinks
Up to 7 fl oz (200 ml) natural unsweetened fruit juice per day (in addition to any suggested in a plan)

There is no alcohol allowance on this plan.

NOTE   1 wholemeal roll should weigh about 2 oz (50 g).
1 slice of wholemeal bread should weigh about 1 oz (25 g).
So, instead of 1 roll you could have 2 slices of bread (or vice versa) if you prefer.

DAY ONE

BREAKFAST	1 oz (25 g) branflakes with skimmed milk from allowance
	1 slice wholemeal toast with low-fat spread from allowance
	1 teaspoon reduced-sugar marmalade or jam
SNACK MEAL	Quick pea soup (*see p. 236*)
	1 wholemeal roll or 2 slices wholemeal bread
	1 small banana or 1 peach
MAIN MEAL	Kedgeree (*see p. 291*)
	Spicy tomato salad (*see p. 323*)
	Strawberry mousse (*see p. 330*)

DAY TWO

BREAKFAST	5 fl oz (150 ml) unsweetened orange juice
	1 Weetabix with skimmed milk from allowance
SNACK MEAL	2 slices wholemeal bread
	2 oz (50 g) roast beef trimmed of all fat cucumber
	1 pear or 4 oz (100 g) strawberries
MAIN MEAL	Spaghetti with fresh tomato and basil sauce (see p. 256)
	Mixed leaf salad (see p. 322) and 1 other salad (see pp. 322–4)
	Oranges in orange jelly (see p. 331)

DAY THREE

BREAKFAST	5 fl oz (150 ml) unsweetened orange juice
	1 oz (25 g) dry oats made into porridge with water or skimmed milk from allowance
	½ chopped banana
SNACK MEAL	Tomato and red pepper soup (see p. 234)
	1 wholemeal roll or 2 slices wholemeal bread
	1 orange or 2 tangerines
MAIN MEAL	Turkeyballs in mushroom and yoghurt sauce (see p. 305)
	2 oz (50 g) pasta shells
	3 oz (75 g) peas
	4 oz (100 g) spinach
	Fruit kebabs (see p. 332)

DAY FOUR

BREAKFAST	4 oz (100 g) unsweetened grapefruit segments 1 slice wholemeal toast and low-fat spread from allowance
SNACK MEAL	2 slices wholemeal bread 2 oz (50 g) corned beef crunchy lettuce 1 pear or 4 oz (100 g) cherries
MAIN MEAL	Grilled trout with bacon (see p. 275) 5 oz (150 g) baked potato 3 oz (75 g) broad beans 4–8 oz (100–225 g) cauliflower Baked apple with sultanas and apple juice (see p. 334)

DAY FIVE

BREAKFAST	1 slice wholemeal toast with low-fat spread from allowance 7 oz (200 g) tin tomatoes
SNACK MEAL	2 slices wholemeal bread 2 oz (50 g) trimmed ham 1 tomato 1 diet yoghurt
MAIN MEAL	Lamb pilaf (see p.320) Button mushroom salad (see p. 322) and 1 other salad (see pp. 322–4) Apple jelly with grapes (see p. 332)

DAY SIX

BREAKFAST	5 fl oz (150 ml) unsweetened orange juice
	1 boiled egg
	1 slice wholemeal toast with low-fat spread from allowance
SNACK MEAL	1 wholemeal roll
	Avgolemono (*see p. 234*)
	1 apple or a slice fresh pineapple
MAIN MEAL	Grilled haddock with fromage frais (*see p. 276*)
	5 oz (150 g) boiled potatoes
	3 oz (75 g) peas
	2 grilled tomatoes
	Baked banana and orange (*see p. 335*)

DAY SEVEN

BREAKFAST	5 fl oz (150 ml) unsweetened apple juice
	1 oz (25 g) unsweetened muesli with skimmed milk from allowance
SNACK MEAL	Salade Niçoise (*see p. 242*)
	1 slice wholemeal bread
	1 diet yoghurt
MAIN MEAL	Ovenbaked crispy chicken made with 4 oz (100 g) chicken (*see p. 296*)
	5 oz (150 g) baked potato
	2 oz (50 g) parsnips
	6 oz (175 g) broccoli
	Pear and tofu whip (*see p. 335*)

DAY EIGHT

BREAKFAST	2 slices wholemeal toast with low-fat spread from allowance 2 teaspoons reduced-sugar marmalade
SNACK MEAL	4 oz (100 g) cottage cheese 2 rye crispbreads 2 tomatoes 1 small banana or 4 oz (100 g) grapes
MAIN MEAL	Prawn and fennel risotto (*see p. 288*) Coleslaw (*see p. 322*) and 1 other salad (*see pp. 322–4*) Strawberries with raspberry sauce (*see p. 336*)

DAY NINE

BREAKFAST	5 fl oz (150 ml) unsweetened orange juice 1 Shredded Wheat with skimmed milk from allowance
SNACK MEAL	2 slices wholemeal bread 2 oz (50 g) skinless cooked chicken breast chopped celery 2 teaspoons low-fat natural yoghurt as dressing 1 diet yoghurt
MAIN MEAL	Grilled cod with parsley sauce (*see p. 276*) (4 oz/100 g) 5 oz (150 g) boiled potatoes 6 oz (175 g) French beans 8 oz (225 g) courgettes Mango cream (*see p. 338*)

DAY TEN

BREAKFAST	1 oz (25 g) branflakes with skimmed milk from allowance
	1 slice wholemeal toast with low-fat spread from allowance
SNACK MEAL	Carrot and dill pâté (see p. 237)
	2 slices wholemeal bread made into Melba toast (see p. 88)
	1 apple or 1 peach or 1 nectarine
MAIN MEAL	Tuna and mushroom supreme (see p. 284)
	2 oz (50 g) bulgar wheat
	2 salads (see pp. 322–4)
	Greek fruit salad (see p. 337)

DAY ELEVEN

BREAKFAST	5 fl oz (150 ml) unsweetened orange juice
	1 oz (25 g) dry oats made into porridge with water or skimmed milk from allowance
	½ chopped banana
SNACK MEAL	Chilled tomato, yoghurt and basil soup (see p. 230)
	1 wholemeal roll or 2 slices wholemeal bread
	1 diet yoghurt
MAIN MEAL	Chicken curry (see p. 297)
	2 oz (50 g) brown rice
	Fresh tomato and onion chutney (see p. 344)
	1 salad (see pp. 322–4)
	Banana split (see p. 336)

DAY TWELVE

BREAKFAST	5 fl oz (150 ml) unsweetened grapefruit juice
	1 oz (25 g) unsweetened muesli with skimmed milk from allowance
SNACK MEAL	2 slices wholemeal bread
	½ tin sardines in brine
	chopped spring onion
	2 teaspoons low-fat natural yoghurt
	4 oz (100 g) raspberries or 4 oz (100 g) strawberries
MAIN MEAL	Quick sweet and sour pork (see p. 308)
	2 oz (50 g) noodles
	6 oz (175 g) broccoli
	1 salad (see pp. 322–4)
	Fresh fruit salad (see p. 338)

DAY THIRTEEN

BREAKFAST	5 fl oz (150 ml) unsweetened orange juice
	1 boiled egg and 1 slice wholemeal toast
SNACK MEAL	Herb and cheese-stuffed tomatoes (see p. 247)
	1 wholemeal roll
	1 diet yoghurt
MAIN MEAL	Spaghetti with broccoli (see p. 255)
	Button mushroom salad (see p. 322)
	1 other salad (see pp. 322–4)
	Orange or apple blancmange (see p. 341)

DAY FOURTEEN

BREAKFAST	7 oz (200 g) tin tomatoes
	1 slice wholemeal toast
SNACK MEAL	2 slices wholemeal bread
	1 oz (25 g) low-fat (14%) Cheddar
	1 teaspoon tomato or Branston pickle
	1 small banana or 3 plums
MAIN MEAL	Cottage cheese and chive omelette
	(*see p. 251*)
	5 oz (150 g) baked potato
	2 salads (*see pp. 322–4*)
	Dried fruit salad (*see p. 337*)

11 The Short, Sharp Shock

(1000 calories a day)

The Short, Sharp Shock provides the lowest number of calories you should go down to for safe and yet quick and effective weight loss. Anyone can use this plan for rapid results but all men and women of average height and who are quite active, will achieve satisfactory weight loss on the other plans. This one is mainly for women of below average height or who are very inactive. However, once you're losing weight steadily, you could try alternating with one of the other plans.

Look through the recipes to decide whether you prefer this plan to the Quickfire Plan (see p. 108). They have the same calorie counts, but this plan is based on more traditional, slightly plainer food than the Quickfire.

Remember the plan is completely flexible. The set plan isn't a magic formula. There's no need to eat chicken on Tuesday or tuna on Thursday if you don't feel like it, or if it's inconvenient. You can interchange any of the meals for an equivalent one. Remember, though, that variety of food is important for a nutritious diet.

You can have your snack meal in the evening instead of at lunchtime if it is easier. Remember, too, that you don't have to eat anything that's on the plan if you're feeling full!

These are the additional allowances for the Short, Sharp Shock (these are sometimes mentioned in the plans but, of course, you may use them as and when you like):

Daily allowance   10 fl oz (300 ml) skimmed milk
Weekly allowance   3 oz (75 g) low-fat spread

Other drinks:
Unlimited tap, still or carbonated water
Unlimited no-cal drinks
Up to 7 fl oz (200 ml) natural unsweetened fruit juice
per day (in addition to any suggested in a plan)

There is no alcohol allowance on this plan.

NOTE   1 wholemeal roll should weigh about 2 oz (50 g).
1 slice of wholemeal bread should weigh about
1 oz (25 g).
So, instead of 1 roll you could have 2 slices of
bread (or vice versa) if you prefer.

DAY ONE

BREAKFAST	1 oz (25 g) branflakes with skimmed milk from allowance
	1 slice wholemeal toast with low-fat spread from allowance
SNACK MEAL	5 fl oz (150 ml) Garden vegetable soup (*see p. 233*)
	2 cream crackers
	2 oz (50 g) Edam or Brie cheese
	1 small banana or 1 peach
MAIN MEAL	Smoky fish pie (*see p. 279*)
	2 oz (50 g) carrots or broccoli
	2 oz (50 g) peas or courgettes
	1 slice wholemeal bread with low-fat spread from allowance
	1 diet yoghurt

DAY TWO

BREAKFAST	5 fl oz (150 ml) unsweetened orange juice 1 Weetabix with skimmed milk from allowance
SNACK MEAL	2 slices wholemeal bread 2 oz (50 g) roast beef trimmed of all fat crunchy lettuce 1 pear or 4 oz (100 g) strawberries
MAIN MEAL	Beef casserole (*see p. 316*) 2 oz (50 g) green beans 1 apple or 4 oz (100 g) cherries

DAY THREE

BREAKFAST	5 fl oz (150 ml) unsweetened orange juice 1 oz (25 g) dry oats made into porridge with water or skimmed milk from allowance 2 oz (50 g) chopped banana
SNACK MEAL	5–7 oz (150–200 g) jacket potato 4 oz (100 g) cottage cheese 1 orange or 2 tangerines
MAIN MEAL	Tuna pasta ribbons (*see p. 287*) 1 diet yoghurt with 4 oz (100 g) chopped apple

DAY FOUR

BREAKFAST	4 oz (100 g) unsweetened grapefruit segments
	2 slices wholemeal toast with low-fat spread from allowance
SNACK MEAL	2 oz (50 g) corned beef
	2 slices wholemeal bread
	crunchy lettuce
	1 pear or 4 oz (100 g) cherries
MAIN MEAL	Quick sweet and sour pork (*see p. 308*)
	2 oz (50 g) brown rice
	green salad (without dressing) or any salad on p. 188
	Spicy pear and orange (*see p. 333*)

DAY FIVE

BREAKFAST	4 oz (100 g) unsweetened grapefruit segments
	2 oz (50 g) unsweetened prunes
	1 slice wholemeal toast with low-fat spread from allowance
SNACK MEAL	Tuna pot rice (*see p. 244*)
	1 diet yoghurt
MAIN MEAL	Grilled chicken rosemary (*see p. 293*)
	5–7 oz (150–200 g) jacket potato
	2 oz (50 g) sliced green beans
	4 oz (100 g) Fresh fruit salad (*see p. 338*)

DAY SIX

BREAKFAST	1 slice lean back bacon, trimmed of all fat and grilled 4 oz (100 g) tinned tomatoes 1 slice wholemeal toast with low-fat spread from allowance
SNACK MEAL	4 oz (100 g) cottage cheese 2 rye crispbreads 2 small tomatoes 1 diet yoghurt
MAIN MEAL	Spanish omelette (*see p. 250*) 2 oz (50 g) mushrooms poached in skimmed milk from allowance 1 slice wholemeal bread with low-fat spread from allowance Baked banana and orange (*see p. 335*)

DAY SEVEN

BREAKFAST	5 fl oz (150 ml) unsweetened orange juice 1 boiled egg 1 slice wholemeal toast with low-fat spread from allowance
SNACK MEAL	2 slices wholemeal bread 2 oz (50 g) trimmed ham 1 small tomato 1 small banana or 4 oz (100 g) grapes
MAIN MEAL	4 oz (100 g) roast leg of lamb trimmed of all fat 5–7 oz (150–200 g) jacket potato 2 oz (50 g) peas or cauliflower 2 oz (50 g) swede or spinach Chopped apple crunch (*see p. 334*)

DAY EIGHT

BREAKFAST	5 fl oz (150 ml) unsweetened apple juice
	1½ oz (40 g) unsweetened muesli with skimmed milk from allowance
SNACK MEAL	Leek and carrot soup (*see p. 232*)
	1 hard-boiled egg
	2 rye crispbreads
	crunchy lettuce
	1 apple or 1 slice fresh pineapple
MAIN MEAL	Chilli mince (*see p. 315*)
	small crusty roll
	green salad (without dressing) or any salad from the 'free' list on p. 188
	4 oz (100 g) Fresh fruit salad (*see p. 338*)

DAY NINE

BREAKFAST	5 fl oz (150 ml) unsweetened orange juice
	1 Weetabix with skimmed milk from allowance
SNACK MEAL	5–7 oz (150–200 g) jacket potato
	2 oz (50 g) chopped ham, trimmed of all fat
	2 oz (50 g) mushrooms poached in skimmed milk from allowance
	1 diet yoghurt with 4 oz (100 g) chopped pear or 4 oz (100 g) whole strawberries
MAIN MEAL	Crunchy fish bake (*see p. 280*)
	4 oz (100 g) baked tomatoes
	2 oz (50 g) peas or leeks
	Baked banana and orange (*see p. 335*)

DAY TEN

BREAKFAST	1 oz (25 g) dry oats made with water or skimmed milk from allowance
	2 oz (50 g) chopped banana
	1 slice wholemeal toast with low-fat spread from allowance
SNACK MEAL	2 slices wholemeal bread
	2 oz (50 g) Edam or Camembert cheese
	1 small tomato
	1 large orange or 4 oz (100 g) raspberries
MAIN MEAL	Fresh mixed herb omelette (see p. 252)
	5–7 oz (150–200 g) jacket potato
	2 oz (50 g) green beans or courgettes
	1 diet yoghurt

DAY ELEVEN

BREAKFAST	4 oz (100 g) unsweetened grapefruit segments
	2 oz (50 g) prunes
	1 slice wholemeal toast with low-fat spread from allowance
SNACK MEAL	4 oz (100 g) cottage cheese
	4 oz (100 g) celery
	2 oz (50 g) carrots
	2 rye crispbreads
	1 apple or peach
MAIN MEAL	Spicy chicken with apple (see p. 295)
	2 oz (50 g) brown rice
	green salad (without dressing) or any 'free' salad on p. 188
	4 oz (100 g) stewed pear
	2 oz (50 g) vanilla ice-cream

DAY TWELVE

BREAKFAST	5 fl oz (150 ml) unsweetened grapefruit juice 1 slice wholemeal toast with low-fat spread from allowance
SNACK MEAL	1 slice wholemeal bread 2 oz (50 g) liver pâté 1 medium tomato 1 small banana or 3 plums
MAIN MEAL	Grilled cod with parsley sauce (*see p. 276*) 5–7 oz (150–200 g) jacket potato 2 oz (50 g) peas 1 diet yoghurt

DAY THIRTEEN

BREAKFAST	1 Shredded Wheat with skimmed milk from allowance 2 oz (50 g) chopped banana
SNACK MEAL	5–7 oz (150–200 g) jacket potato 2 small low-fat sausages, grilled 4 oz (100 g) tinned tomatoes 1 pear
MAIN MEAL	Macaroni cottage cheese (*see p. 257*) green salad (without dressing) or any 'free' salad on p. 188 1 slice wholemeal toast 4 oz (100 g) Fresh fruit salad (*see p. 338*)

DAY FOURTEEN

BREAKFAST   5 fl oz (150 ml) unsweetened orange
            juice
            1 egg scrambled in a non-stick pan with
            1 tablespoon skimmed milk from
            allowance
            1 slice wholemeal toast with low-fat
            spread from allowance

SNACK MEAL 2 slices wholemeal bread
            2 oz (25 g) mashed sardines
            cucumber
            1 diet yoghurt

MAIN MEAL   4 oz (100 g) roast chicken, with the skin
            removed
            5–7 oz (150–200 g) baked potato
            2 oz (50 g) peas
            2 oz (50 g) carrots or leeks
            Spicy pear and orange (*see p. 333*)

12 The Middle Way

(1250 calories a day)

This plan is designed so that most women (unless they're of very small build or very inactive) will lose weight on it at a very satisfactory rate. All men will quickly lose weight on it.

Look through the recipes to decide whether you prefer this plan to The Easy Way (see p. 135). They have the same calorie counts, but this plan is based on more traditional, slightly plainer food than The Easy Way.

Remember the plan is completely flexible. The set plan isn't a magic formula. There's no need to eat chicken on Tuesday or tuna on Thursday if you don't feel like it, or if it's inconvenient. You can interchange any of the meals for an equivalent one. Remember, though, that variety of food is important for a nutritious diet.

You can have your snack meal in the evening instead of at lunchtime if it is easier. Remember, too, that you don't have to eat everything on the plan if you're feeling full!

These are the additional allowances for The Middle Way (these are sometimes mentioned in the plans but, of course, you may use them as and when you like):

Daily allowance   10 fl oz (300 ml) skimmed milk
Weekly allowance 3 oz (75 g) low-fat spread

Other drinks
Unlimited tap, still or carbonated water
Unlimited no-cal drinks
Up to 7 fl oz (200 ml) natural unsweetened fruit juice
per day (in addition to any suggested in a plan)

Optional:
1 alcoholic drink per day, choosing from:
1 glass wine
½ pint beer *or* cider *or* lager
1 small sherry *or* port *or* martini
1 single measure of spirits such as whisky *or* gin with
slimline mixer

Remember, it's not compulsory to have the alcoholic
drink! If you don't drink it, you'll lose weight a little
more quickly.

NOTE   1 wholemeal roll should weigh about 2 oz (50 g).
1 slice of wholemeal bread should weigh about
1 oz (25 g).
So, instead of 1 roll you could have 2 slices of
bread (or vice versa) if you prefer.

DAY ONE

BREAKFAST	5 fl oz (150 ml) unsweetened orange juice 2 Weetabix with skimmed milk from allowance
SNACK MEAL	2 slices wholemeal bread 2 oz (50 g) mashed sardines cucumber and cress 1 diet yoghurt
MAIN MEAL	6 oz (175 g) gammon steak, grilled pineapple ring 2 oz (50 g) sweetcorn or peas 4 oz (100 g) baked tomato Baked banana and orange (*see p. 335*)

DAY TWO

BREAKFAST	4 oz (100 g) unsweetened grapefruit segments 2 slices wholemeal toast with low-fat spread from allowance
SNACK MEAL	4 oz (100 g) low-fat burger, grilled lettuce, tomato and/or onion wholemeal bun 1 apple
MAIN MEAL	Chilli mince (*see p. 315*) 2 oz (50 g) brown rice 4 oz (100 g) Fresh fruit salad (*see p. 338*) 2 oz (50 g) vanilla ice-cream

DAY THREE

BREAKFAST	5 fl oz (150 ml) unsweetened apple juice
	2 oz (50 g) unsweetened muesli with
	skimmed milk from allowance
SNACK MEAL	2 slices wholemeal bread
	2 oz (50 g) roast chicken
	crunchy lettuce
	1 small tomato
	1 pear or 4 oz (100 g) strawberries
MAIN MEAL	Spanish omelette (*see p. 250*)
	2 oz (50 g) mushrooms poached in
	skimmed milk from allowance
	5 oz (150 g) tinned tomatoes
	1 slice wholemeal bread with low-fat
	spread from allowance
	1 diet yoghurt

DAY 4

BREAKFAST	1 oz (25 g) branflakes with skimmed
	milk from allowance
	1 slice wholemeal toast with low-fat
	spread from allowance
SNACK MEAL	2 slices wholemeal bread
	2 oz (50 g) low-fat Cheddar or Edam
	finely chopped onion
	1 diet yoghurt
MAIN MEAL	Beef casserole (*see p. 316*)
	7–9 oz (200–250 g) jacket potato
	2 oz (50 g) carrots or green beans
	Chopped apple crunch (*see p. 334*)

DAY FIVE

BREAKFAST	5 fl oz (150 ml) unsweetened orange juice
	1 oz (25 g) dry oats made into porridge with water or skimmed milk from allowance
	2 oz (50 g) chopped banana
	1 slice wholemeal toast with low-fat spread from allowance
SNACK MEAL	Tuna pot rice (see p. 244)
	1 diet yoghurt
MAIN MEAL	Grilled chicken rosemary (see p. 293)
	Ratatouille (see p. 344)
	4 oz (100 g) boiled, sliced potatoes
	Spicy pear and orange (see p. 333)

DAY SIX

BREAKFAST	2 rashers lean back bacon, trimmed of all fat and grilled
	5 oz (125 g) tinned tomatoes
	1 slice wholemeal toast
SNACK MEAL	5 oz (150 g) reduced-sugar baked beans
	2 slices wholemeal toast
	1 diet yoghurt
MAIN MEAL	Sardine and tomato pizza (see p. 283)
	green salad (without dressing) or any salad from the 'free' list on p. 188
	7–9 oz (200–250 g) jacket potato
	1 apple or 4 oz (100 g) strawberries

DAY SEVEN

BREAKFAST	5 fl oz (150 ml) unsweetened orange juice
	1 boiled egg
	1 slice wholemeal toast with low-fat spread from allowance
SNACK MEAL	2 slices wholemeal bread
	2 oz (50 g) lean ham
	1 small tomato
	1 small banana or 4 oz (100 g) grapes
MAIN MEAL	4 oz (100 g) skinless roast chicken
	7–9 oz (200–250 g) jacket potato
	2 oz (50 g) peas or courgettes
	2 oz (50 g) carrots or cabbage
	1 teaspoon stuffing and gravy
	Baked apple with sultanas and apple juice (*see p. 334*)

DAY EIGHT

BREAKFAST	1 Shredded Wheat with milk from allowance
	1 slice wholemeal toast with low-fat spread from allowance
SNACK MEAL	5 fl oz (150 ml) Garden vegetable soup (*see p. 233*)
	wholemeal roll
	1 oz (25 g) low-fat Cheddar or Edam
	1 orange or tangerine
MAIN MEAL	4 oz (100 g) lean lamb chop and rosemary, grilled
	8 oz (225 g) boiled potatoes with skin on
	4 oz (100 g) baked tomatoes
	2 oz (50 g) peas or leeks
	4 oz (100 g) chopped apple or strawberries and 1 diet yoghurt

DAY NINE

BREAKFAST	5 fl oz (150 ml) unsweetened orange juice
	1 oz (25 g) branflakes with skimmed milk from allowance
	2 oz (50 g) chopped banana
SNACK MEAL	7–9 oz (200–250 g) jacket potato
	2 oz (50 g) tuna
	cucumber
	1 pear
MAIN MEAL	Beef and vegetable curry (see p. 311)
	2 oz (50 g) brown rice
	wholemeal roll
	tomato and onion salad (made with 2 small tomatoes)
	2 oz (50 g) vanilla ice-cream

DAY TEN

BREAKFAST	4 oz (100 g) unsweetened grapefruit segments
	2 oz (50 g) unsweetened prunes
	2 slices wholemeal toast with low-fat spread from allowance
SNACK MEAL	2 slices wholemeal bread
	cucumber
	2 oz (50 g) cottage cheese
	1 small banana or 4 oz (100 g) raspberries
MAIN MEAL	Tuna pasta ribbons (see p. 287)
	1 slice wholemeal bread
	Chopped apple crunch (see p. 334)

DAY ELEVEN

BREAKFAST	5 fl oz (150 ml) unsweetened orange juice
	2 Weetabix with skimmed milk from allowance
SNACK MEAL	2 slices wholemeal bread
	2 oz (50 g) lean roast beef
	crunchy lettuce
	1 small tomato
	1 pear
MAIN MEAL	Smoky fish pie (see p. 279)
	2 oz (50 g) carrots or broccoli
	2 oz (50 g) peas or leeks
	wholemeal roll
	2 oz (50 g) sliced banana or strawberries and 1 diet yoghurt

DAY TWELVE

BREAKFAST	5 fl oz (150 ml) unsweetened orange juice
	1 oz (25 g) dry oats made into porridge with water or skimmed milk from allowance
	2 oz (50 g) banana
	1 slice wholemeal toast with low-fat spread from allowance
SNACK MEAL	2 slices wholemeal bread
	2 oz (50 g) corned beef
	crunchy lettuce
	1 orange
MAIN MEAL	Chicken and vegetable rice (see p. 301)
	wholemeal roll
	green salad (with 1 tablespoon dressing on p. 325) or any 'free' salad on p. 208
	4 oz (100 g) Fresh fruit salad (see p. 338)

DAY THIRTEEN

BREAKFAST	5 fl oz (150 ml) unsweetened orange juice
	1 egg scrambled in a non-stick pan with 1 tablespoon skimmed milk from allowance
	1 slice wholemeal toast with low-fat spread from allowance
SNACK MEAL	4 oz (100 g) low-fat burger, grilled lettuce, tomato and/or onion wholemeal bun
	1 apple
MAIN MEAL	Macaroni cottage cheese (see p. 257)
	1 rasher lean back bacon, trimmed of all fat and grilled
	1 slice wholemeal toast
	Spicy pear and orange (see p. 333)

DAY FOURTEEN

BREAKFAST	4 oz (100 g) unsweetened grapefruit segments
	2 slices wholemeal toast with low-fat spread from allowance
SNACK MEAL	2 slices wholemeal bread
	1 hard-boiled egg finely chopped with onion and cress
	1 apple
MAIN MEAL	4 oz (100 g) lean roast lamb and mint sauce
	7–9 oz (200–250 g) jacket potato
	2 oz (50 g) cabbage or leeks
	2 oz (50 g) swede or green beans
	Baked banana and orange (see p. 335)

13 The Easy Way

(1250 calories a day)

This plan is designed so that most women (unless they're of very small build or very inactive) will lose weight on it at a very satisfactory rate. All men will quickly lose weight on it.

Look through the recipes to decide whether you prefer this plan to The Middle Way (see p. 126). They have the same calorie counts, but this plan is based on more modern, slightly fancier food than The Middle Way.

Remember the plan is completely flexible. The set plan isn't a magic formula. There's no need to eat chicken on Tuesday or tuna on Thursday if you don't feel like it, or if it's inconvenient. You can interchange any of the meals for an equivalent one. Remember, though, that variety of food is important for a nutritious diet.

You can have your snack meal in the evening instead of at lunchtime if it is easier. Remember, too, that you don't have to eat everything that's on the plan if you're feeling full!

These are the additional allowances for The Easy Way (these are sometimes mentioned in the plans but, of course, you may use them as and when you like):

Daily allowance 10 fl oz (300 ml) skimmed milk
Weekly allowance 3 oz (75 g) low-fat spread

Other drinks:
Unlimited tap, still or carbonated water
Unlimited no-cal drinks
Up to 7 fl oz (200 ml) natural unsweetened fruit juice
per day (in addition to any suggested in a plan)

Optional:
1 alcoholic drink per day, choosing from:
1 glass wine
½ pint beer *or* cider *or* lager
1 small sherry *or* port *or* martini
1 single measure of spirits such as whisky *or* gin with
slimline mixer

Remember, it's not compulsory to have the alcoholic
drink! If you don't drink it, you'll lose weight a little
more quickly.

NOTE 1 wholemeal roll should weigh about 2 oz (50 g).
    1 slice of wholemeal bread should weigh about
    1 oz (25 g).
    So, instead of 1 roll you could have 2 slices of
    bread (or vice versa) if you prefer.

Breakfast every week day
2 oz (50 g) unsweetened muesli with skimmed milk from
allowance and with a choice of chopped fresh fruit: apple,
pear, tangerine, some grapes, a banana or some dried fruit,
soaked then cooked and cooled, e.g. apricots or prunes.
Coffee or tea, with skimmed milk from allowance if you
wish but no sugar.

Breakfasts at weekends
5 fl oz (150 ml) unsweetened orange juice

Choice of:
Small grilled or microwaved kipper
Smoked haddock fillet, poached in skimmed milk from allowance
Tinned tomatoes on wholemeal toast or sliced fresh tomatoes, grilled, on wholemeal toast
Coffee or tea with skimmed milk from allowance if you wish but no sugar.

DAY ONE

SNACK MEAL	2 slices wholemeal bread with low-fat spread from allowance 2 oz (50 g) cold sliced roast chicken, with skin removed watercress 1 teaspoon low-fat yoghurt as dressing 1 piece fresh fruit
MAIN MEAL	3 oz (75 g) roast chicken breast, sliced with skin removed 5 oz (150 g) new potatoes 3 oz (75 g) broad beans 3 oz (75 g) carrots gravy – as fat free as possible Apricot fool (*see p. 339*)

DAY TWO

SNACK MEAL	2 slices wholemeal bread with low-fat spread from allowance 2 oz (50 g) chicken tomato and cucumber 1 piece fresh fruit
MAIN MEAL	Chick pea paprika (*see p. 266*) 2–3 oz (50–75 g) brown rice 1 diet yoghurt

DAY THREE

SNACK MEAL	2 slices wholemeal bread with low-fat spread from allowance ½ tin sardines in brine, drained sliced pickled dill cucumber 1 piece fresh fruit
MAIN MEAL	Chicken Provençale (*see p. 294*) 5–7 oz (150–200 g) baked potato mixed salad: lettuce, endive, radicchio, Chinese leaves, etc., with Yoghurt, lemon and herb dressing (*see p. 325*) Fresh fruit salad (*see p. 338*)

DAY FOUR

SNACK MEAL 2 slices wholemeal bread with low-fat
spread from allowance
2 oz (50 g) lean boiled ham (visible fat
removed)
French mustard
1 piece fresh fruit

MAIN MEAL Tagliatelle al limone (*see p. 236*)
tomato and spring onion salad made
with 3 small tomatoes with Yoghurt,
lemon and herb dressing
(*see p. 325*)
5 oz (150 g) low-fat natural yoghurt
mixed with 1 small mashed banana
2 teaspoons sultanas

DAY FIVE

SNACK MEAL 2 slices wholemeal bread with low-fat
spread from allowance
1½ oz (40 g) low-fat Cheddar-type
cheese
1 teaspoon tomato pickle
1 piece fresh fruit

MAIN MEAL Tuna and bulgar risotto (*see p. 286*)
salad made with 1 head chicory and 1
orange, dressed with low-fat natural
yoghurt and orange juice
1 piece fresh fruit

DAY SIX

SNACK MEAL 2 slices wholemeal bread with low-fat
spread from allowance
2 oz (50 g) tuna in brine or water, drained
1 tomato, sliced
1 piece fresh fruit

MAIN MEAL Stir-fry beef and noodles (see p. 312)
5 oz (150 g) low-fat natural yoghurt mixed
with 1 fresh segmented tangerine or
satsuma

DAY SEVEN

SNACK MEAL 2-egg fresh herb omelette (parsley, chives
and tarragon)
1 slice wholemeal bread
1 piece fresh fruit

MAIN MEAL Stuffed sardines (see p. 282)
5–7 oz (150–200 g) baked potato with low
fat spread from allowance
3 oz (75 g) peas
Pineapple fool (see p. 339)

DAY EIGHT

SNACK MEAL Pasta shapes in tomato sauce (see p. 258)
1 piece fresh fruit

MAIN MEAL Veal al limone (see p. 309)
5 oz (150 g) new potatoes
mixed salad: lettuce, radicchio, grated carrot
strips of red pepper with Yoghurt, lemon
and herb dressing (see p. 325)
4–6 oz (100–175 g) Fresh fruit salad (see p. 338) with 1 tablespoon 1% fromage frais

DAY NINE

SNACK MEAL   2 slices wholemeal bread with low-fat
spread from allowance
½ tin mackerel in brine with 2 teaspoons low-fat natural yoghurt and 1
teaspoon of capers
1 piece fresh fruit

MAIN MEAL   Chinese fish and noodles (*see p. 280*)
1 piece fresh fruit

DAY TEN

SNACK MEAL   2 slices wholemeal bread with low-fat
spread from allowance
1 oz (25 g) pastrami
sliced dill cucumber
1 low-fat fruit yoghurt

MAIN MEAL   Chicken Provençale (*see p. 294*)
5–7 oz (150–200 g) baked potato
3 oz (75 g) sweetcorn
1 piece fresh fruit

DAY ELEVEN

SNACK MEAL   2 slices wholemeal bread with low-fat
spread from allowance
1½ oz (40 g) smoked pork loin
1 teaspoon apricot chutney
1 piece fresh fruit

MAIN MEAL   Tuna cassoulet (*see p. 285*)
salad of lettuce, Chinese leaves and
watercress, Yoghurt, lemon and herb
dressing (*see p. 325*)
Baked apple with sultanas and apple
juice (*see p. 334*)

DAY TWELVE

SNACK MEAL	2 slices wholemeal bread with low-fat spread from allowance 2 slices back bacon trimmed of all fat and grilled lettuce and tomato – as much as you can fit on! 1 teaspoon low-fat natural yoghurt as dressing 1 low-fat fruit yoghurt
MAIN MEAL	Chicken and bulgar risotto made with brown rice (*see p. 286*) tomato and spring onion salad made with 3 small tomatoes with Yoghurt, lemon and herb dressing (*see p. 325*) 1 piece fresh fruit

DAY THIRTEEN

SNACK MEAL	2 slices wholemeal toast topped with 8 oz (225 g) reduced-sugar baked beans 1 piece fresh fruit
MAIN MEAL	1 × 6–7 oz (175–200 g) grilled trout 1 teaspoon Dijon mustard mixed with 1 tablespoon low-fat natural yoghurt as a sauce 5 oz (150 g) new potatoes 3 oz (75 g) frozen spinach, cooked and 1 tablespoon fromage frais, stirred in off the heat Passion fruit fool (*see p. 339*)

DAY FOURTEEN

SNACK MEAL | 5–7 oz (150–200 g) baked potato with low-fat spread from allowance
¼ oz (10 g) grated low-fat Cheddar cheese
1 tablespoon chopped spring onions
1 piece fresh fruit

MAIN MEAL | Pasta with creamy mushrooms
(see p. 259)
mixed salad of lettuce, tomatoes, cucumber and grated carrot with Yoghurt, lemon and herb dressing (see p. 325)
4–6 oz (100–175 g) Fresh fruit salad (see p. 338)

14 The Vegetarian Plan

(1250 calories a day)

This plan is designed so that most women (unless they're of very small build or very inactive) will lose weight on it at a very satisfactory rate. All men will quickly lose weight on it.

It's designed to appeal to all vegetarians and others who feel like having a change from meat- or fish-based dishes.

Remember the plan is completely flexible. The set plan isn't a magic formula. There's no need to eat chick peas on Tuesday or pizza on Thursday if you don't feel like it, or if it's inconvenient. You can interchange any of the meals for an equivalent one. Remember, though, that variety of food is important for a nutritious diet.

You can have your snack meal in the evening instead of at lunchtime if it is easier. Remember, too, that you don't have to eat everything that's on the plan if you're feeling full!

There's a flexible version of this diet plan on p. 190 where you will find a lot more choice for breakfast, snack meals and main meals.

These are the additional allowances for The Vegetarian Plan (these are sometimes mentioned in the plans but, of course, you may use them as and when you like):

Daily allowance   10 fl oz (300 ml) skimmed milk
Weekly allowance 3 oz (75 g) low-fat spread

Other drinks:
Unlimited tap, still or carbonated water
Unlimited no-cal drinks
Up to 7 fl oz (200 ml) natural unsweetened fruit juice
per day (in addition to any suggested in a plan)

Optional:
1 alcoholic drink per day, choosing from:
1 glass wine
½ pint beer or cider or lager
1 small sherry or port or martini
1 single measure of spirits such as whisky or gin with
slimline mixer

Remember, it's not compulsory to have the alcoholic
drink! If you don't drink it, you'll lose weight a little
more quickly.

NOTE   1 wholemeal roll should weigh about 2 oz (50 g).
       1 slice of wholemeal bread should weigh about
       1 oz (25 g).
       So, instead of 1 roll you could have 2 slices of
       bread (or vice versa) if you prefer.

For vegetarians the following may also be helpful:
* If you prefer, you can substitute vegetarian Cheddar for
  any recipes which specify Parmesan cheese.
* Agar agar can be substituted for the gelatine in any of the
  recipes.
* For any recipe using chicken stock, you can use vegetable stock instead.

DAY ONE

BREAKFAST	5 fl oz (150 ml) unsweetened orange juice
	2 Weetabix with skimmed milk from allowance
SNACK MEAL	Cottage cheese and chive omelette (*see p. 251*)
	1 wholemeal roll or 2 slices wholemeal bread
	1 apple
MAIN MEAL	Mushroom risotto (*see p. 260*)
	Tomato salad and 1 other salad (*see pp. 322–4*)
	The BBC Diet chocolate mousse (*see p. 329*)

DAY TWO

BREAKFAST	4 oz (100 g) unsweetened grapefruit segments
	2 slices wholemeal toast with low-fat spread from allowance
	2 teaspoons reduced-sugar jam or marmalade
SNACK MEAL	Baked potato with Arab salad and cottage cheese (*see p. 245*)
	1 pear
MAIN MEAL	Vegetable stir-fry (*see p. 266*)
	2½ oz (65 g) brown rice
	2 salads (*see pp. 322–4*)
	Oranges in orange jelly (*see p. 331*)

DAY THREE

BREAKFAST	5 fl oz (150 ml) unsweetened apple juice 2 oz (50 g) unsweetened muesli with skimmed milk from allowance
SNACK MEAL	Roasted pepper salad (see p. 239) 1 wholemeal roll or 2 slices wholemeal bread 1 diet yoghurt
MAIN MEAL	Chick pea curry (½ quantity) (see p. 264) and 2 oz (50 g) (dry weight) brown rice Minty cucumber salad (see p. 323) and 1 other salad (see pp. 322–4) Strawberry mousse (see p. 330)

DAY FOUR

BREAKFAST	1 oz (25 g) branflakes and 5 fl oz (150 ml) skimmed milk from allowance 1 slice wholemeal toast with low-fat spread from allowance 1 teaspoon reduced-sugar jam or marmalade
SNACK MEAL	Mushrooms à la Grecque (see p. 240) 1 wholemeal roll 1 peach
MAIN MEAL	Frittata (see p. 252) Mixed leaf salad (see p. 322) and 1 other salad (see pp. 322–4) Fruit kebabs (see p. 332)

DAY FIVE

BREAKFAST	5 fl oz (150 ml) unsweetened orange juice 1 oz (25 g) dry oats made into porridge with water or skimmed milk from allowance 1 slice wholemeal toast with low-fat spread from allowance 1 teaspoon reduced-sugar jam or marmalade
SNACK MEAL	Gazpacho (*see p. 231*) 2 slices wholemeal bread 4 oz (100 g) strawberries
MAIN MEAL	Cauliflower cheese (*see p. 264*) Arab salad (*see p. 322*) and 1 other salad (*see pp. 322–4*) Baked apple with sultanas and apple juice (*see p. 334*)

DAY SIX

BREAKFAST	7 oz (200 g) tin tomatoes on 1 slice wholemeal toast or grilled fresh tomatoes on 1 slice wholemeal toast 1 piece of fresh fruit
SNACK MEAL	Carrot and dill pâté (*see p. 237*) 2 slices wholemeal bread or toast 3 plums
MAIN MEAL	Barbecued tofu with rice (*see p. 263*) 2½ oz (65 g) brown rice 2 salads (*see pp. 322–4*) Apple jelly with grapes (*see p. 332*)

DAY SEVEN

BREAKFAST
5 fl oz (150 ml) unsweetened orange juice
1 boiled egg
1 slice wholemeal bread or toast
1 piece of fresh fruit

SNACK MEAL
Herb and cheese-stuffed tomatoes (see p. 247)
1 wholemeal roll
2 satsumas or 2 tangerines

MAIN MEAL
Pasta with creamy mushrooms (see p. 259)
Spicy tomato salad (see p. 323) and 1 other salad (see pp. 322–4)
Baked banana and orange (see p. 335)

DAY EIGHT

BREAKFAST
1 Shredded Wheat with skimmed milk from allowance
1 slice wholemeal toast with low-fat spread from allowance
1 teaspoon reduced-sugar jam or marmalade

SNACK MEAL
Chilled cucumber and mint soup (see p. 230)
2 slices wholemeal bread
4 oz (100 g) grapes

MAIN MEAL
Vegetable chilli (see p. 269)
Coleslaw (see p. 322) and 1 other salad (see pp. 322–4)
Slimmers' lemon cheesecake (see p. 340)

DAY NINE

BREAKFAST	5 fl oz (150 ml) unsweetened grapefruit juice
	1 oz (25 g) branflakes with skimmed milk from allowance
	½ chopped banana
SNACK MEAL	Greek salad (*see p. 241*)
	1 wholemeal roll
	1 diet fruit fromage frais
MAIN MEAL	Broccoli risotto (*see p. 260*)
	Tomato salad (*see p. 322*) and 1 other salad (*see pp. 322–4*)
	Pear and tofu whip (*see p. 335*)

DAY TEN

BREAKFAST	2 oz (50 g) unsweetened prunes and 2 oz (50 g) unsweetened grapefruit
	1 slice wholemeal toast with low-fat spread from allowance
	1 teaspoon reduced-sugar marmalade
SNACK MEAL	Quick bean soup (*see p. 235*)
	1 wholemeal roll
	1 small banana
MAIN MEAL	Mushroom, olive and caper pizza (*see p. 268*)
	Mixed leaf salad and 1 other salad (*see pp. 322–4*)
	Strawberries with raspberry sauce (*see p. 336*)

DAY ELEVEN

BREAKFAST	4 oz (100 g) 'dry-fried' mushrooms (*see p. 86*) 1 slice wholemeal toast with low-fat spread from allowance
SNACK MEAL	Hummus (*see p. 238*) 1 slice wholemeal bread or 1 wholemeal pitta bread 1 peach
MAIN MEAL	Peppers stuffed with bulgar pilaf (*see p. 270*) Arab salad (*see p. 322*) and 1 other salad (*see pp. 322–4*) Mango cream (*see p. 338*)

DAY TWELVE

BREAKFAST	5 fl oz (150 ml) unsweetened orange juice 1 egg scrambled in a non-stick pan with 1 tablespoon skimmed milk from allowance 1 grilled tomato 1 slice wholemeal toast with low-fat spread from allowance
SNACK MEAL	Courgettes à la Grecque (*see p. 241*) 1 wholemeal roll 4 oz (100 g) raspberries
MAIN MEAL	Potato and mushroom gratin (*see p. 262*) 6 oz (175 g) steamed broccoli 6 oz (175 g) carrots Apple cinnamon toast (*see p. 330*)

DAY THIRTEEN

BREAKFAST	5 fl oz (150 ml) unsweetened grapefruit juice
	2 oz (50 g) unsweetened muesli with skimmed milk from allowance
SNACK MEAL	Chilled tomato, yoghurt and basil soup (*see p. 230*)
	1 wholemeal roll
	4 oz (100 g) cherries
MAIN MEAL	Fresh mixed herb omelette (*see p. 252*)
	7 oz (200 g) baked potato with low-fat spread from allowance or low-fat natural yoghurt
	6 oz (175 g) French beans
	4 oz (100 g) spinach
	Banana split (*see p. 336*)

DAY FOURTEEN

BREAKFAST	5 fl oz (150 ml) unsweetened orange juice
	1 boiled egg
	1 slice wholemeal toast with low-fat spread from allowance
SNACK MEAL	Cottage cheese and fruit salad (*see p. 248*)
	2 slices wholemeal bread
	1 diet yoghurt
MAIN MEAL	Vegetarian moussaka (*see p. 271*)
	Spicy tomato salad (*see p. 323*)
	1 other salad (*see pp. 322–4*)
	Fresh fruit salad (*see p. 338*)

15 The Gourmet Plan

(1250 calories a day)

This plan is designed so that most women (unless they're of very small build or very inactive) will lose weight on it at a very satisfactory rate. All men will quickly lose weight on it.

It's for those who love their food and want to eat really tempting meals while they lose weight.

Remember the plan is completely flexible. The set plan isn't a magic formula. There's no need to eat chicken on Tuesday or tuna on Thursday if you don't feel like it, or if it's inconvenient. You can interchange any of the meals for an equivalent one. Remember, though, that variety of food is important for a nutritious diet.

You can have your snack meal in the evening instead of at lunchtime if it is easier. Remember, too, that you don't have to eat everything that's on the plan if you're feeling full!

There's a flexible version of this diet plan on p. 199 where you will find a lot more choice for breakfast, snack meals and main meals.

These are the additional allowances for The Gourmet Plan (these are sometimes mentioned in the plans but, of course, you may use them as and when you like):

THE COMPLETE BBC DIET

Daily allowance   10 fl oz (300 ml) skimmed milk
Weekly allowance   3 oz (75 g) low-fat spread

Other drinks:
Unlimited tap, still or carbonated water
Unlimited no-cal drinks
Up to 7 fl oz (200 ml) natural unsweetened fruit juice
per day (in addition to any suggested in a plan)

Optional:
1 alcoholic drink per day, choosing from:
1 glass wine
½ pint beer *or* cider *or* lager
1 small sherry *or* port *or* martini
1 single measure of spirits such as whisky *or* gin with
slimline mixer

Remember, it's not compulsory to have the alcoholic
drink! If you don't drink it, you'll lose weight a little
more quickly.

NOTE   1 wholemeal roll should weigh about 2 oz (50 g).
        1 slice of wholemeal bread should weigh about
        1 oz (25 g).
        So, instead of 1 roll you could have 2 slices of
        bread (or vice versa) if you prefer.

DAY ONE

BREAKFAST 5 fl oz (150 ml) unsweetened orange juice
2 Weetabix with skimmed milk from allowance

SNACK MEAL Avgolemono (*see p. 234*)
1 wholemeal roll or 2 slices wholemeal bread
1 apple

MAIN MEAL Pork escalopes with white wine (*see p. 307*)
Potato gratin using 7 oz (200 g) potatoes (*see p. 342*)
6 oz (175 g) steamed broccoli
6 oz (175 g) carrots
The BBC Diet chocolate mousse (*see p. 329*)

DAY TWO

BREAKFAST 4 oz (100 g) unsweetened grapefruit segments
2 slices wholemeal toast with low-fat spread from allowance
2 teaspoons reduced-sugar jam or marmalade

SNACK MEAL Tapénade (*see p. 237*)
2 slices wholemeal bread or toast
1 diet yoghurt

MAIN MEAL Lamb and mint kebabs with yoghurt sauce (*see p. 317*)
2 oz (50 g) brown rice
Arab salad (see p. 322) and 1 other salad (*see pp. 322–4*)
Baked apple with sultanas and apple juice (*see p. 334*)

DAY THREE

BREAKFAST	5 fl oz (150 ml) unsweetened apple juice
	1½ oz (40 g) unsweetened muesli with skimmed milk from allowance
SNACK MEAL	Tomato and red pepper soup (see p. 234)
	1 wholemeal roll or 2 slices wholemeal bread
	4 oz (100 g) raspberries
MAIN MEAL	Stir-fried beef and broccoli (see p. 313)
	3 oz (75 g) noodles
	2 salads (see pp. 322–4)
	Strawberry mousse (see p. 330)

DAY FOUR

BREAKFAST	1 oz (25 g) branflakes with skimmed milk from allowance
	1 teaspoon reduced-sugar jam or marmalade
SNACK MEAL	Greek salad (see p. 241)
	1 wholemeal roll or 2 slices wholemeal bread
	3 fresh figs
MAIN MEAL	Turkey 'saltimbocca' (see p. 302)
	7 oz (200 g) baked potato
	4 oz (100 g) spinach
	3 oz (75 g) broad beans
	Baked banana and orange (see p. 335)

DAY FIVE

BREAKFAST	5 fl oz (150 ml) unsweetened orange juice 1 oz (25 g) dry oats made into porridge with water or milk from allowance 1 slice wholemeal toast with low-fat spread from allowance 1 teaspoon reduced-sugar jam or marmalade
SNACK MEAL	Salade Niçoise (*see p. 242*) 1 wholemeal roll or 2 slices of wholemeal bread 4 oz (100 g) grapes
MAIN MEAL	Trout with cucumber sauce (*see p. 275*) 7 oz (200 g) boiled potatoes 3 oz (75 g) mangetout 2 grilled tomatoes Strawberries with raspberry sauce (*see p. 336*)

DAY SIX

BREAKFAST	7 oz (200 g) tin tomatoes 1 slice wholemeal toast or grilled fresh tomatoes on 1 slice wholemeal toast
SNACK MEAL	Tabbouleh (*see p. 243*) unlimited salad from 'free' list on p. 208 1 pear
MAIN MEAL	Monkfish provençale (*see p. 290*) 2½ oz (65 g) brown rice 4 oz (100 g) courgettes 4 oz (100 g) 'dry-fried' mushrooms (*see p. 86*) Banana split (*see p. 336*)

DAY SEVEN

BREAKFAST	5 fl oz (150 ml) unsweetened orange juice
	1 boiled egg
	1 slice wholemeal bread or toast
SNACK MEAL	Quick gravad lax (see p. 249)
	unlimited salad from 'free' list (see p. 208)
	2 slices wholemeal bread
	3 apricots
MAIN MEAL	Roast chicken with fresh herbs (with 3 oz/75 g skinless breast, see p. 300)
	7 oz (200 g) boiled potatoes
	6 oz (175 g) French beans
	6 oz (175 g) swede
	Orange or apple blancmange (see p. 341)

DAY EIGHT

BREAKFAST	1 Shredded Wheat with skimmed milk from allowance
	1 slice wholemeal toast with low-fat spread from allowance
	1 teaspoon reduced-sugar jam or marmalade
SNACK MEAL	Baked potato with crispy bacon and Arab salad filling (see p. 246)
	1 low-fat diet fruit fromage frais
MAIN MEAL	Marinated lamb cutlets (see p. 319)
	7 oz (200 g) boiled potatoes
	3 oz (76 g) peas
	5 oz (150 g) leeks
	Fruit kebabs (see p. 332)

DAY NINE

BREAKFAST	5 fl oz (150 ml) unsweetened grapefruit juice
	1 oz (25 g) branflakes with skimmed milk from allowance
SNACK MEAL	Tuna-stuffed pitta (*see p. 244*)
	4 oz (100 g) raspberries
MAIN MEAL	Haddock with yellow pepper sauce (*see p. 277*)
	2½ oz (65 g) brown rice
	6 oz (175 g) French beans
	4–8 oz (100–225 g) cauliflower
	Slimmers' lemon cheesecake (*see p. 340*)

DAY TEN

BREAKFAST	2 oz (50 g) unsweetened prunes
	2 slices wholemeal toast with low-fat spread from allowance
	2 teaspoons reduced-sugar jam or marmalade
SNACK MEAL	Gazpacho (*see p. 231*)
	1 wholemeal roll or 2 slices wholemeal bread
	1 pear
MAIN MEAL	Calf's or lamb's liver with orange and vermouth (*see p. 310*)
	7 oz (200 g) boiled new potatoes
	6 oz (175 g) broccoli
	3 oz (75 g) broad beans
	Apple jelly with grapes (*see p. 332*)

DAY ELEVEN

BREAKFAST	4 oz (100 g) 'dry-fried' mushrooms (*see p. 86*) 1 slice wholemeal toast with low-fat spread from allowance
SNACK MEAL	Roasted pepper salad (*see p. 239*) 1 wholemeal roll 2 satsumas or 2 mandarins or 2 tangerines
MAIN MEAL	Turkey kebabs marinated in yoghurt, lime and ginger (*see p. 304*) 2½ oz (65 g) bulgar wheat Spicy tomato salad (*see p. 323*) and 1 other salad (*see pp. 322–4*) Apple cinnamon toast (*see p. 330*)

DAY TWELVE

BREAKFAST	5 fl oz (150 ml) unsweetened orange juice 1 egg scrambled in a non-stick pan with 1 tablespoon skimmed milk from allowance 1 grilled tomato 1 slice wholemeal toast with low-fat spread from allowance
SNACK MEAL	Quick bean soup (*see p. 235*) 1 wholemeal roll or 2 slices wholemeal bread 1 slice melon (any variety)
MAIN MEAL	Stuffed baked trout (*see p. 273*) 7 oz (200 g) baked potato Coleslaw (*see p. 322*) Oranges in orange jelly (*see p. 331*)

DAY THIRTEEN

BREAKFAST   5 fl oz (150 ml) unsweetened grapefruit
                 juice
                 1½ oz (40 g) unsweetened muesli with
                 skimmed milk from allowance
SNACK MEAL   Cold trout marinated in orange
                 (see p. 274)
                 unlimited salad from 'free' list
                 (see p. 208)
                 1 wholemeal roll or 2 slices wholemeal
                 bread
                 1 peach or 1 nectarine
MAIN MEAL   Pasta shells with prawns, lime and dill
                 (see p. 289)
                 Tomato salad (see p. 322) and 1 other
                 salad (see pp. 322–4)
                 Mango cream (see p. 338)

DAY FOURTEEN

BREAKFAST   4 oz (100 g) unsweetened grapefruit
                 segments
                 1 boiled egg
                 1 slice wholemeal bread or toast
SNACK MEAL   Mushrooms à la Grecque (see p. 240)
                 1 wholemeal roll or 2 slices wholemeal
                 bread
                 1 diet yoghurt
MAIN MEAL   Turkey escalopes Marsala (see p. 303)
                 7 oz (200 g) Potatoes baked with lemon
                 and garlic (see p. 343)
                 4 oz (100 g) spinach
                 3 oz (75 g) peas
                 Greek fruit salad (see p. 337)

16 The Slower But Sure Plan

(1500 calories a day)

Most men find they lose weight at a very satisfactory rate with this plan and this will also be the case for most women who also increase their physical activity (see chapter 21).

Look through the recipes to decide whether you prefer this plan to The Hearty-eating Plan (see p. 171). They have the same calorie counts, but this plan is based on more traditional, slightly plainer food than The Hearty-eating Plan.

Remember the plan is completely flexible. The set plan isn't a magic formula. There's no need to eat chicken on Tuesday or tuna on Thursday if you don't feel like it, or if it's inconvenient. You can interchange any of the meals for an equivalent one. Remember, though, that variety of food is important for a nutritious diet.

You can have your snack meal in the evening instead of at lunchtime if it is easier. Remember, too, that you don't have to eat everything that's on the plan if you're feeling full!

These are the additional allowances for The Slower But Sure Plan (these are sometimes mentioned in the plans but, of course, you may use them as and when you like):

Daily allowance   10 fl oz (300 ml) skimmed milk
Weekly allowance 3 oz (75 g) low-fat spread

Other drinks:
Unlimited tap, still or carbonated water
Unlimited no-cal drinks
Up to 7 fl oz (200 ml) natural unsweetened fruit juice
per day (in addition to any suggested in a plan)

Optional:
1 alcoholic drink per day, choosing from:
1 glass wine
½ pint beer *or* cider *or* lager
1 small sherry *or* port *or* martini
1 single measure of spirits such as whisky *or* gin with
slimline mixer

Remember, it's not compulsory to have the alcoholic
drink! If you don't drink it, you'll lose weight a little
more quickly.

NOTE   1 wholemeal roll should weigh about 2 oz (50 g).
        1 slice of wholemeal bread should weigh about
        1 oz (25 g).
        So, instead of 1 roll you could have 2 slices of
        bread (or vice versa) if you prefer.

DAY ONE

BREAKFAST	5 fl oz (150 ml) unsweetened orange juice 2 Weetabix with skimmed milk from allowance 2 slices wholemeal toast with low-fat spread from allowance
SNACK MEAL	3 slices wholemeal bread 3 oz (75 g) lean ham 1 medium tomato 1 large orange or 1 slice fresh pineapple
MAIN MEAL	Chunky vegetables and beef (*see p. 314*) large crusty roll 2 oz (50 g) peas or leeks Spicy pear and orange (*see p. 333*) 4 oz (100 g) vanilla ice-cream

DAY TWO

BREAKFAST	2 eggs scrambled in a non-stick pan with 1 tablespoon skimmed milk from allowance 2 slices wholemeal toast with low-fat spread from allowance
SNACK MEAL	3 slices wholemeal bread 3 oz (75 g) Edam or Brie cheese 2 teaspoons Branston or other pickle 1 apple or 4 oz (100 g) strawberries
MAIN MEAL	4 oz (100 g) gammon, grilled 7–9 oz (200–250 g) jacket potato 2 oz (50 g) peas or leeks 2 oz (50 g) sweetcorn 4 oz (100 g) Fresh fruit salad (*see p. 338*)

DAY THREE

BREAKFAST	1 oz (25 g) branflakes with skimmed milk from allowance 4 oz (100 g) chopped banana 2 slices wholemeal toast with low-fat spread from allowance
SNACK MEAL	7–9 oz (200–250 g) jacket potato 5 oz (150 g) baked beans 1 orange
MAIN MEAL	Spicy chicken with apple (*see p. 295*) 2½ oz (65 g) brown rice tomato and onion salad (made with 2 small tomatoes) Chopped apple crunch (*see p. 334*) 1 diet yoghurt

DAY FOUR

BREAKFAST	5 fl oz (150 ml) unsweetened orange juice 1 oz (25 g) dry oats made into porridge with water or skimmed milk from allowance 4 oz (100 g) chopped banana 2 slices wholemeal toast with low-fat spread from allowance
SNACK MEAL	3 slices wholemeal bread Smoked mackerel pâté cucumber 1 apple or 4 oz (100 g) raspberries
MAIN MEAL	Shepherd's pie (*see p. 316*) 4 oz (100 g) cauliflower or sprouts 3 cream crackers 2 oz (50 g) Edam or Brie cheese

DAY FIVE

BREAKFAST	5 fl oz (150 ml) unsweetened orange juice
	1 Shredded Wheat with skimmed milk from allowance
	2 slices wholemeal toast with low-fat spread from allowance
SNACK MEAL	3 slices wholemeal bread
	3 oz (75 g) lean ham, trimmed of all fat
	1 medium tomato
	1 large orange or 1 slice fresh pineapple
MAIN MEAL	Chilli mince (*see p. 315*)
	2½ oz (65 g) brown rice
	green salad (without dressing) or any salad on p. 217
	4 oz (100 g) Fresh fruit salad (*see p. 338*)
	4 oz (100 g) vanilla ice-cream

DAY SIX

BREAKFAST	2 rashers lean back bacon, trimmed of all fat and grilled
	4 oz (100 g) tinned tomatoes
	2 oz (50 g) mushrooms
	2 slices wholemeal toast with low-fat spread from allowance
SNACK MEAL	3 slices wholemeal bread
	3 oz (75 g) skinless cooked chicken breast
	cucumber
	1 pear or peach
MAIN MEAL	Sardine and tomato pizza (*see p. 283*)
	green salad (without dressing) or any salad on p. 217
	9 oz (250 g) jacket potato
	2 cream crackers
	2 oz (50 g) Edam cheese

DAY SEVEN

BREAKFAST	1 oz (25 g) branflakes with skimmed milk from allowance
	4 oz (100 g) chopped banana
	2 slices wholemeal toast with low-fat spread from allowance
SNACK MEAL	2-egg Fresh mixed herb omelette (*see p. 252*)
	2 slices wholemeal bread with low-fat spread from allowance
	2 medium tomatoes
	1 pear
MAIN MEAL	4 oz (100 g) lean roast lamb
	9 oz (250 g) jacket potato
	3 oz (75 g) peas or 4 oz (100 g) spinach
	3 oz (75 g) cabbage or sprouts
	Chopped apple crunch (*see p. 334*)
	1 diet yoghurt

DAY EIGHT

BREAKFAST	5 fl oz (150 ml) unsweetened orange juice
	1 Shredded Wheat with skimmed milk from allowance
	2 slices wholemeal toast with low-fat spread from allowance
SNACK MEAL	3 slices wholemeal bread
	2 oz (50 g) tuna in brine or water, drained
	lettuce
	1 small banana
MAIN MEAL	Chicken and vegetable rice (*see p. 301*)
	2 cream crackers
	2 oz (50 g) Edam cheese
	2 oz (50 g) vanilla ice-cream

DAY NINE

BREAKFAST	5 fl oz (150 ml) unsweetened orange juice
	2 slices wholemeal toast
	2 oz (50 g) lean back bacon, trimmed of all fat and grilled
SNACK MEAL	9 oz (250 g) jacket potato
	2 oz (50 g) low-fat Cheddar cheese
	1 oz (25 g) onion, chopped
	1 diet yoghurt
MAIN MEAL	Crunchy fish bake (see p. 280)
	8 oz (225 g) boiled/jacket potato
	up to 6 oz (175 g) carrots or unlimited courgettes
	Baked banana and orange (see p. 335)

DAY TEN

BREAKFAST	5 fl oz (150 ml) unsweetened orange juice
	2 Weetabix with skimmed milk from allowance
	2 slices wholemeal toast with low-fat spread from allowance
SNACK MEAL	3 slices wholemeal bread
	3 oz (75 g) lean ham
	1 medium tomato
	1 orange
MAIN MEAL	Beef and vegetable curry (see p. 311)
	2 oz (50 g) brown rice
	2 cream crackers
	2 oz (50 g) Edam cheese
	2 oz (50 g) vanilla ice-cream
	4 oz (100 g) banana or 3 fresh apricots

DAY ELEVEN

BREAKFAST	5 fl oz (150 ml) unsweetened orange juice
	1 oz (25 g) dry oats made into porridge with water or skimmed milk from allowance
	4 oz (100 g) chopped banana
	2 slices wholemeal toast with low-fat spread from allowance
SNACK MEAL	3 slices wholemeal bread
	3 oz (75 g) mashed sardines
	1 medium tomato
	1 pear
MAIN MEAL	Quick sweet and sour pork (*see p. 308*)
	8 oz (225 g) baked potato
	4 oz (100 g) Fresh fruit salad (*see p. 338*)
	2 oz (50 g) vanilla ice-cream

DAY TWELVE

BREAKFAST	5 fl oz (150 ml) unsweetened orange juice
	1 Shredded Wheat with skimmed milk from allowance
	2 slices wholemeal toast with low-fat spread from allowance
SNACK MEAL	3 slices wholemeal bread
	3 oz (75 g) Edam cheese
	1 medium tomato
	1 apple
MAIN MEAL	Tuna pasta ribbons (*see p. 287*)
	1 slice wholemeal bread
	1 diet yoghurt

DAY THIRTEEN

BREAKFAST
: 2 rashers lean back bacon, trimmed of all fat and grilled
1 small low-fat sausage, grilled
4 oz (100 g) tinned tomatoes
1 slice wholemeal toast with low-fat spread from allowance

SNACK MEAL
: Mushroom omelette (*see p. 250*)
2 slices wholemeal bread with low-fat spread from allowance
2 medium tomatoes
1 pear

MAIN MEAL
: Calf's or lamb's liver with orange and vermouth (*see p. 310*)
2½ oz (65 g) brown rice
2 oz (50 g) peas or leeks
4 oz (100 g) vanilla ice-cream

DAY FOURTEEN

BREAKFAST
: 1 oz (25 g) branflakes with skimmed milk from allowance
4 oz (100 g) chopped banana
2 slices wholemeal toast with low-fat spread from allowance

SNACK MEAL
: 7 oz (200 g) tin reduced-sugar baked beans
2 slices wholemeal toast
1 diet yoghurt

MAIN MEAL
: 4 oz (100 g) skinless roast chicken
7–9 oz (200–250 g) boiled potatoes
2 oz (50 g) peas or unlimited courgettes
2 oz (50 g) carrots or broccoli
1 tablespoon stuffing and gravy
Baked apple with sultanas and apple juice (*see p. 334*)

17 The Hearty-eating Plan

(1500 calories a day)

Most men find they lose weight at a very satisfactory rate with this plan and this will also be the case for most women who also increase their physical activity (see chapter 21).

Look through the recipes to decide whether you prefer this plan to The Slower But Sure Plan (see p. 162). They have the same calorie counts, but this plan is based on more modern, slightly fancier food than The Slower But Sure.

Remember the plan is completely flexible. The set plan isn't a magic formula. There's no need to eat chicken on Tuesday or tuna on Thursday if you don't feel like it, or if it's inconvenient. You can interchange any of the meals for an equivalent one. Remember, though, that variety of food is important for a nutritious diet.

You can have your snack meal in the evening instead of at lunchtime if it is easier. Remember, too, that you don't have to eat everything that's on the plan if you're feeling full!

There's a flexible version of this diet plan on p. 210 where you will find a lot more choice for breakfast, snack meals and main meals.

These are the additional allowances for The Hearty-eating Plan (these are sometimes mentioned in the plans but, of course, you may use them as and when you like):

Daily allowance   10 fl oz (300 ml) skimmed milk
Weekly allowance 3 oz (75 g) low-fat spread

Other drinks:
Unlimited tap, still or carbonated water
Unlimited no-cal drinks
Up to 7 fl oz (200 ml) natural unsweetened fruit juice
per day (in addition to any suggested in a plan)

Optional:
1 alcoholic drink per day, choosing from:
1 glass wine
½ pint beer or cider or lager
1 small sherry or port or martini
1 single measure of spirits such as whisky or gin with
slimline mixer

Remember, it's not compulsory to have the alcoholic
drink! If you don't drink it, you'll lose weight a little
more quickly.

NOTE   1 wholemeal roll should weigh about 2 oz (50 g).
           1 slice of wholemeal bread should weigh about
           1 oz (25 g).
           So, instead of 1 roll you could have 2 slices of
           bread (or vice versa) if you prefer.

DAY ONE

BREAKFAST	5 fl oz (150 ml) unsweetened orange juice
	2 Weetabix with skimmed milk from allowance
	1 slice wholemeal toast with low-fat pread from allowance
	1 teaspoon reduced-sugar jam or marmalade
SNACK MEAL	Quick pea soup (see p. 236)
	1 wholemeal roll or 2 slices wholemeal bread
	1 apple and 1 pear
MAIN MEAL	Turkey burgers (see p. 306)
	7–9 oz (200–250 g) baked potato
	Tomato salad (see p. 322) and 1 other salad (see pp. 322–4)
	Slimmers' lemon cheesecake (see p. 340)

DAY TWO

BREAKFAST	5 fl oz (150 ml) unsweetened orange juice
	2 rashers lean back bacon, trimmed of all fat and grilled
	1 grilled tomato
	2 slices wholemeal toast with low-fat spread from allowance
SNACK MEAL	Potato and leek soup (see p. 232)
	1 wholemeal roll or 2 slices wholemeal bread
	1 peach and 4 oz (100 g) grapes
MAIN MEAL	Sardine fishcakes (see p. 281)
	8 oz (225 g) cauliflower
	6 oz (175 g) carrots
	Strawberry mousse (see p. 330)

DAY THREE

BREAKFAST	2 rashers lean back bacon, trimmed of fat and grilled
	1 small low-fat sausage, grilled
	1 grilled tomato
	1 slice wholemeal toast with low-fat spread from allowance
SNACK MEAL	Salade Niçoise (*see p. 242*)
	1 wholemeal roll or 2 slices wholemeal bread
	1 small banana and 1 diet yoghurt
MAIN MEAL	Lamb's kidneys in mushroom sauce (*see p. 318*)
	3 oz (75 g) brown rice
	6 oz (175 g) broccoli
	4 oz (100 g) spinach
	Baked apple with sultanas and apple juice (*see p. 334*)

DAY FOUR

BREAKFAST	2 poached eggs
	2 slices wholemeal toast with low-fat spread from allowance
SNACK MEAL	Gazpacho (*see p. 231*)
	1 wholemeal roll or 2 slices wholemeal bread
	1 peach and 4 oz (100 g) raspberries
MAIN MEAL	Lamb-stuffed peppers (*see p. 321*)
	Coleslaw (*see p. 322*) and 1 other salad (*see p. 322–4*)
	Banana split (*see p. 336*)

DAY FIVE

BREAKFAST   5 fl oz (150 ml) unsweetened grapefruit
juice
2 oz (50 g) dry oats made into porridge
with water or milk from allowance
1 small banana

SNACK MEAL   Courgettes à la Grecque (*see p. 241*)
2 slices wholemeal bread
4 oz (100 g) cherries and 1 diet yoghurt

MAIN MEAL   Ovenbaked crispy chicken (*see p. 296*)
7–9 oz (200–250 g) boiled new potatoes
2 grilled tomatoes
4 oz (100 g) broad beans
Dried fruit salad (*see p. 337*)

DAY SIX

BREAKFAST   5 fl oz (150 ml) unsweetened orange juice
1 boiled egg
2 slices of wholemeal toast with low-fat
spread from allowance

SNACK MEAL   3 slices wholemeal bread with low-fat
spread from allowance
3 oz (75 g) ham, trimmed of all fat
2 tomatoes and other salads from 'free'
list (*see p. 218*)
1 small banana and 1 orange

MAIN MEAL   Steak with mustard sauce (*see p. 314*)
Potatoes baked with lemon and garlic (*see
p. 343*) using 7–9 oz (200–250 g) potatoes
4 oz (100 g) 'dry-fried' mushrooms
(*see p. 86*)
3 oz (75 g) broad beans
Apple jelly with grapes (*see p. 332*)

DAY SEVEN

BREAKFAST	5 oz (150 g) unsweetened apple juice
	2 Shredded Wheat with skimmed milk from allowance
	1 slice wholemeal toast with low-fat spread from allowance
SNACK MEAL	Greek salad (see p. 241)
	2 slices wholemeal bread
	3 apricots and 3 fresh figs
MAIN MEAL	Chicken in barbecue sauce (see p. 292)
	7–9 oz (200–250 g) baked potato
	Arab salad (see p. 322) and 1 other salad (see pp. 322–4)
	Strawberries with raspberry sauce (see p. 336)

DAY EIGHT

BREAKFAST	5 fl oz (150 ml) unsweetened orange juice
	7 oz (200 g) tin tomatoes
	2 slices wholemeal toast with low-fat spread from allowance
SNACK MEAL	7–9 oz (200–250 g) Baked potato with crispy bacon and Arab salad filling (see p. 246)
	1 apple and 4 oz (100 g) cherries
MAIN MEAL	Fisherman's pie (see p. 278)
	6 oz (175 g) carrots
	5 oz (150 g) leeks
	Mango cream (see p. 338)

DAY NINE

BREAKFAST   5 fl oz (150 ml) unsweetened grapefuit juice
1 small grilled kipper
1 slice wholemeal toast with low-fat spread
from allowance

SNACK MEAL   2 slices wholemeal bread with low-fat
spread from allowance
2 oz (50 g) low-fat (14%) Cheddar
2 teaspoons Branston or tomato pickle
1 pear and 1 slice melon

MAIN MEAL   4 oz (100 g) grilled gammon steak,
trimmed of all fat
7–9 oz (200–250 g) baked potato
2 grilled tomatoes
3 oz (75 g) peas
Orange or apple blancmange (*see p. 341*)

DAY TEN

BREAKFAST   4 oz (100 g) unsweetened grapefruit
segments
5 oz (150 g) smoked haddock fillet,
poached
1 slice wholemeal toast with low-fat spread
from allowance

SNACK MEAL   Quick bean soup (*see p. 235*)
1 wholemeal roll or 2 slices wholemeal
bread
1 slice fresh pineapple and 1 diet yoghurt

MAIN MEAL   Chicken stir-fry (*see p. 294*)
3 oz (75 g) brown rice
1 salad (*see pp. 322–4*)
Oranges in orange jelly (*see p. 331*)

DAY ELEVEN

BREAKFAST	5 fl oz (150 ml) unsweetened orange juice
	2 Weetabix with skimmed milk from allowance
	1 slice wholemeal toast with low-fat spread from allowance
SNACK MEAL	3 slices wholemeal bread
	3 oz (75 g) corned beef
	2 teaspoons Piccalilli
	3 plums and 1 apple
MAIN MEAL	4 oz (100 g) lean leg roast lamb with 2 tablespoons gravy (made with most of fat removed)
	7–9 oz (200–250 g) boiled new potatoes
	4–8 oz (100–225 g) spring cabbage
	6 oz (175 g) carrots
	Fruit kebabs (see p. 332)

DAY TWELVE

BREAKFAST	2 poached eggs
	2 slices wholemeal toast with low-fat spread from allowance
SNACK MEAL	Hummus (see p. 238)
	2 slices wholemeal bread or toast
	1 orange and 1 peach
MAIN MEAL	Mixed grill of 2 trimmed back rashers bacon (2 oz/50 g)
	2 small low-fat sausages
	2 grilled tomatoes
	4 oz (100 g) grilled or 'dry-fried' mushrooms (see p. 86)
	2 slices wholemeal bread
	Baked banana and orange (see p. 335)

DAY THIRTEEN

BREAKFAST	5 fl oz (150 ml) unsweetened grapefruit juice 2 oz (50 g) dry oats made into porridge with water and skimmed milk from llowance 1 small banana
SNACK MEAL	Tuna-stuffed potato (*see recipe and* NOTE *p. 246*) using 7–9 oz (200–250 g) potato 2 diet yoghurts
MAIN MEAL	Quick stir-fried pork with beansprouts (*see p. 308*) 3 oz (75 g) noodles 2 salads (*see pp. 322–4*) Pear and tofu whip (*see p. 335*)

DAY FOURTEEN

BREAKFAST	5 fl oz (150 ml) unsweetened orange juice 2 rashers of lean back bacon, trimmed of fat and grilled 1 grilled tomato 2 slices wholemeal toast with low-fat spread from allowance
SNACK MEAL	3 slices wholemeal bread 3 oz (75 g) roast beef trimmed of all fat tomato, cucumber and lettuce or other salad from the 'free' list (*see p. 218*) 4 oz (100 g) strawberries and 1 apple
MAIN MEAL	Roast chicken with mushrooms, with 4 oz (100 g) skinless breast (*see p. 298*) 7 oz (200 g) boiled new potatoes 6 oz (175 g) French beans 4 oz (100 g) spinach *The BBC Diet* chocolate mousse (*see p. 329*)

18 The Flexible Plans

(1000 calories a day)

For a more flexible version of The Quickfire Plan choose one breakfast, one snack meal and one main meal (plus pudding) for each day. You'll see that there are also guidelines for what to eat with your main meal in the way of potatoes, rice, vegetables etc.

Remember, your additional allowances are as follows (sometimes mentioned in the lists but, of course, to be used as and when you like):

Daily allowance   10 fl oz (300 ml) skimmed milk
Weekly allowance   3 oz (75 g) low-fat spread

Other drinks:
Unlimited tap, still or carbonated water
Unlimited no-cal drinks
Up to 7 fl oz (200 ml) natural unsweetened fruit juice per day (in addition to any suggested in a plan)

There is no alcohol allowance on this plan.

NOTE   1 wholemeal roll should weigh about 2 oz (50 g).
1 slice of wholemeal bread should weigh about 1 oz (25 g). So, instead of 1 roll you could have 2 slices of bread (or vice versa) if you prefer.

BREAKFASTS

Choose any breakfast from:

1   1 oz (25 g) branflakes with skimmed milk from
    allowance
    1 slice wholemeal toast with low-fat spread from
    allowance
    1 teaspoon reduced-sugar jam or marmalade

2   5 fl oz (150 ml) unsweetened orange juice
    1 oz (25 g) dry oats made into porridge with water
    or skimmed milk from allowance
    ½ chopped banana

3   5 fl oz (150 ml) unsweetened orange juice
    1 Weetabix with skimmed milk from allowance

4   4 oz (100 g) unsweetened grapefruit segments
    1 slice wholemeal toast with low-fat spread from
    allowance
    1 teaspoon reduced-sugar jam or marmalade

5   7 oz (200 g) tin tomatoes
    1 slice wholemeal toast

6   Grilled fresh tomatoes
    1 slice wholemeal toast

7   5 fl oz (150 ml) unsweetened orange juice
    1 boiled egg
    1 slice wholemeal bread or toast with low-fat spread
    from allowance

8   5 fl oz (150 ml) unsweetened apple juice
    1 oz (25 g) unsweetened muesli with skimmed milk
    from allowance

9   2 slices wholemeal toast with low-fat spread from allowance
     2 teaspoons reduced-sugar jam or marmalade ·

10   5 fl oz (150 ml) unsweetened grapefruit juice
     1 Shredded Wheat with skimmed milk from allowance

11   2 pieces fresh fruit
     1 diet yoghurt

12   Fresh fruit salad (*see p. 338*) or tinned fruit in natural juice
     low-fat yoghurt

13   4 oz (100 g) 'dry-fried' mushrooms (*see p. 86*)
     1 slice wholemeal toast

14   3 pieces fresh fruit

SNACK MEALS

Choose one item from list A and one from list B:

Snack meal A

1   Quick pea soup (*see p. 236*)
    wholemeal roll or 2 slices wholemeal bread

2   2 slices wholemeal bread
    2 oz (50 g) roast beef trimmed of all fat
    cucumber, lettuce, tomato, spring onion

3   Tomato and red pepper soup (*see p. 234*)
    1 wholemeal roll or 2 slices wholemeal bread

4   2 slices wholemeal bread
    2 oz (50 g) corned beef
    crunchy lettuce or any other salad from 'free' list on p. 188

5   2 slices wholemeal bread
    2 oz (50 g) ham trimmed of all fat
    tomato or any other salad from 'free' list on p. 188

6   Avgolemono (*see p. 234*)
    1 wholemeal roll or 2 slices wholemeal bread

7   Salade Niçoise (*see p. 242*)
    1 wholemeal roll or 2 slices of wholemeal bread

8   2 slices wholemeal bread
    2 oz (50 g) skinless cooked chicken breast
    chopped celery
    2 teaspoons low-fat natural yoghurt

9   4 oz (100 g) cottage cheese
    2 rye crispbreads
    2 tomatoes, piece of cucumber

10 Carrot and dill pâté (*see p. 237*)
    2 slices wholemeal bread made into Melba toast
    (*see p. 88*)

11 Chilled tomato, yoghurt and basil soup (*see p. 230*)
    1 wholemeal roll or 2 slices wholemeal bread

12 2 slices wholemeal bread
    ½ tin sardines in brine
    any salads from 'free' list on p. 188

13 2 slices wholemeal bread
    2 oz (50 g) low-fat (14%) Cheddar or
    1 oz (40 g) Edam
    1 teaspoon tomato or Branston pickle

14 Herb and cheese-stuffed tomatoes (*see p. 247*)
    1 wholemeal roll or 2 slices wholemeal bread

15 2 slices wholemeal bread
    2 oz (50 g) tuna in brine or water
    any salad from 'free' list on p. 188

16   2 slices wholemeal bread
     2 oz (50 g) salmon in brine or water
     any salad from 'free' list on p. 188

17   2 slices wholemeal bread
     2 oz (50 g) prawns
     2 teaspoons low-fat natural yoghurt
     thick cucumber slices

18   8 oz (225 g) baked beans
     2 slices wholemeal toast

19   2 oz (50 g) crab (fresh, frozen or tinned)
     any 2 salads from 'free' list on p. 188
     1 wholemeal roll or 2 slices wholemeal bread

20   Cottage cheese and chive omelette (see p. 251)

21   Baked potato (5 oz/150 g) with Arab salad and
     cottage cheese filling (see p. 245)

22   Roasted pepper salad (see p. 239)
     1 wholemeal roll or 2 slices wholemeal bread

23   Mushrooms à la Grecque (see p. 240)
     1 wholemeal roll or 2 slices wholemeal bread

24   Gazpacho (see p. 231)
     1 wholemeal roll or 2 slices wholemeal bread

25   Chilled cucumber and mint soup (see p. 230)
     1 wholemeal roll or 2 slices wholemeal bread

26   Hummus (see p. 238)
     2 slices wholemeal bread made into Melba toast
     (see p. 88) or 1 wholemeal pitta bread

27   Cottage cheese and fruit salad (see p. 248)
     2 slices wholemeal bread

28   Courgettes à la Grecque (see p. 241)
     1 wholemeal roll or 2 slices wholemeal bread

29 Tuna omelette (*see p. 284*)
    1 wholemeal roll or 2 slices wholemeal bread

30 Tapénade (*see p. 237*)
    2 slices wholemeal bread made into Melba toast
    (*see p. 88*)

Snack meal B

Any fruit can be accompanied by unlimited low-fat natural
yoghurt or as much 1% fromage frais as you like.

1   1 apple
2   1 pear
3   1 small banana
4   1 orange
5   2 satsumas or 2 tangerines
6   4 oz (100 g) grapes
7   4 oz (100 g) cherries
8   1 peach
9   1 nectarine
10 3 apricots
11 3 plums
12 2 fresh figs
13 Large slice melon
14 Large slice watermelon
15 Large slice fresh pineapple
16 4 oz (100 g) strawberries
17 4 oz (100 g) raspberries
18 1 diet yoghurt, any flavour
19 1 low-fat diet fromage frais, any flavour
20 4 oz (100 g) any fruit tinned in natural juice.
    Choose from: apricot halves, fruit salad, grapefruit
    segments, mandarins, peaches, pears, pineapple,
    raspberries, strawberries

MAIN MEALS

Choose any main meal from the following list, then see below for a choice of accompaniments. Finally, choose a pudding!

1 Kedgeree (*see p. 291*)
2 Spaghetti with fresh tomato and basil sauce (*see p. 256*)
3 Turkeyballs in mushroom and yoghurt sauce (*p. 305*)
4 Grilled trout with bacon (*see p. 275*)
5 Lamb pilaf (*see p. 320*)
6 Grilled haddock with fromage frais (*see p. 276*)
7 Ovenbaked crispy chicken (*see p. 296*)
8 Prawn and fennel risotto (*see p. 288*)
9 Grilled cod with parsley sauce (*see p. 276*)
10 Tuna and mushroom supreme (*see p. 284*)
11 Chicken curry (*see p. 297*) with Fresh tomato and onion chutney (*see p. 344*)
12 Quick sweet and sour pork (*see p. 308*)
13 Spaghetti with broccoli (*see p. 255*)
14 Tuna omelette (*see p. 284*)
15 Cottage cheese and chive omelette (*see p. 251*)
16 Plain grilled trout (6 oz/175 g)
17 Grilled cod or haddock (5 oz/150 g)
18 Cauliflower cheese (*see p. 264*)
19 Vegetable stir-fry (*see p. 266*)
20 Fresh mixed herb omelette (*see p. 252*)

If your main meal dish already includes rice, potatoes, pasta, noodles or bulgar wheat choose one item from list **B** and one from list **C**. (Alternatively you can pick two items from list **B** *or* two from list **C**.)

If your dish does not include rice, potatoes etc., then

choose one item from list **A**, one from **B** and one from **C**. (Again, you can pick two from list **B** *or* two from **C** if you prefer.)

Main meal A

5 oz (150 g) baked potato
5 oz (150 g) boiled potatoes
Potato gratin with 5 oz (150 g) potato (*see p. 342*)
Potato baked with lemon and garlic with 5 oz (150 g) potato (*see p. 343*)
2 oz (50 g) pasta
2 oz (50 g) noodles
2 oz (50 g) bulgar wheat
2 oz (50 g) brown rice

Main meal B

Up to:

3 oz (75 g) broad beans
6 oz (175 g) French beans
6 oz (175 g) Brussels sprouts
8 oz (225 g) cabbage
6 oz (175 g) broccoli
6 oz (175 g) carrots
8 oz (225 g) kale
5 oz (150 g) leeks
2 oz (50 g) parsnips
3 oz (75 g) peas
4 oz (100 g) spinach
6 oz (175 g) swede
8 oz (225 g) turnips
2 oz (50 g) sweetcorn

Or, as much as you like of the following 'free' list:

cauliflower
celery
Chinese cabbage
chicory

courgettes
marrow
mushrooms

All vegetables to be boiled, 'dry-fried' (see p. 86), steamed or microwaved. Do not add any fat during the cooking method or while eating them.

Main meal C

Unlimited quantities except where indicated.

Tomato salad (see p. 322)
Arab salad (see p. 322)
Coleslaw (see p. 322)
Button mushroom salad (see p. 322)
Spicy tomato salad (see p. 323)
Minty cucumber salad (see p. 323)
Roasted pepper salad (see p. 239)
Pea salad with 3 oz (75 g) peas (see p. 324)
Broad bean salad with 3 oz (75 g) broad beans (see p. 324)
Mangetout salad with 3 oz (75 g) mangetout (see p. 324)
Fennel and red pepper salad (see p. 323)

Or, have limited quantities of the following 'free' list salad vegetables with, if you like, either 1 tablespoon of low-fat mayonnaise (see p. 346) or 1 quantity of any salad dressing on pp. 325–8:

alfalfa sprouts
beansprouts
carrots, grated
beansprouts
celery
Chinese leaves
cucumber
endive

chicory
lettuce (all kinds)
mustard and cress
peppers
radishes
tomatoes
watercress

MAIN MEAL PUDDINGS

Choose any pudding from:

1 Strawberry mousse (*see p. 330*)
2 Oranges in orange jelly (*see p. 331*)
3 Apple jelly with grapes (*see p. 332*)
4 Fruit kebabs (*see p. 332*)
5 Baked apple with sultanas and apple juice
   (*see p. 334*)
6 Baked banana and orange (*see p. 335*)
7 Pear and tofu whip (*see p. 335*)
8 Banana split (*see p. 336*)
9 Strawberries with raspberry sauce (*see p. 336*)
10 Greek fruit salad (*see p. 337*)
11 Fresh fruit salad (*see p. 338*)
12 Dried fruit salad (*see p. 337*)
13 Mango cream (*see p. 338*)
14 Orange or apple blancmange (*see p. 341*)

THE FLEXIBLE VEGETARIAN PLAN

(1250 calories a day)

For a more flexible version of The Vegetarian Plan choose one breakfast, one snack meal and one main meal (plus pudding) for each day. You'll see that there are also guidelines for what to eat with your main meal in the way of potatoes, rice, vegetables etc.

Remember, your additional allowances are as follows (sometimes mentioned in the lists but, of course, to be used as and when you like):

Daily allowance   10 fl oz (300 ml) skimmed milk
Weekly allowance   3 oz (75 g) low-fat spread

Other drinks:
Unlimited tap, still or carbonated water
Unlimited no-cal drinks
Up to 7 fl oz (200 ml) natural unsweetened fruit juice per day (in addition to any suggested in a plan)

Optional:
1 alcoholic drink per day, choosing from:
1 glass wine
½ pint beer or cider or lager
1 small sherry or port or martini
1 single measure of spirits such as whisky or gin with slimline mixer

Remember, if you don't have the alcoholic drink you'll lose weight a little more quickly.

NOTE   1 wholemeal roll should weigh about 2 oz (50 g).
        1 slice of wholemeal bread should weigh about
        1 oz (25 g). So, instead of 1 roll you could have 2
        slices of bread (or vice versa) if you prefer.

BREAKFASTS

Choose any breakfast from:

1   5 fl oz (150 ml) unsweetened orange juice
    2 Weetabix with skimmed milk from allowance

2   4 oz (100 g) unsweetened grapefruit segments
    2 slices wholemeal toast with low-fat spread from
    allowance
    2 teaspoons reduced-sugar jam or marmalade

3   5 fl oz (150 ml) unsweetened apple juice
    2 oz (50 g) unsweetened muesli with skimmed milk
    from allowance

4   1 oz (25 g) branflakes with skimmed milk from
    allowance
    1 slice wholemeal toast with low-fat spread from
    allowance
    1 teaspoon reduced-sugar jam or marmalade

5   5 oz (150 ml) unsweetened orange juice
    1 oz (25 g) dry oats made into porridge with water
    or skimmed milk from allowance
    1 slice wholemeal toast with low-fat spread from
    allowance
    1 teaspoon reduced-sugar jam or marmalade

6   7 oz (200 g) tin tomatoes on 1 slice wholemeal toast
    or grilled fresh tomatoes on 1 slice wholemeal toast
    1 piece of fresh fruit

7   5 fl oz (150 ml) unsweetened orange juice
    1 boiled egg
    1 slice wholemeal bread or toast
    1 piece of fresh fruit

8 1 Shredded Wheat with skimmed milk from
   allowance
   1 slice wholemeal toast with low-fat spread from
   allowance
   1 teaspoon reduced-sugar jam or marmalade

9 5 fl oz (150 ml) unsweetened grapefruit juice
   1 oz (25 g) branflakes with skimmed milk from
   allowance
   ½ chopped banana

10 2 oz (50 g) unsweetened prunes and 2 oz (50 g)
   unsweetened grapefruit
   1 slice wholemeal toast with low-fat spread from
   allowance
   1 teaspoon reduced-sugar marmalade

11 4 oz (100 g) mushrooms, 'dry-fried' (see p. 86)
   1 slice wholemeal toast with low-fat spread from
   allowance

12 5 fl oz (150 ml) unsweetened orange juice
   1 egg scrambled in a non-stick pan with 1 tablespoon skimmed milk from allowance
   1 grilled tomato
   1 slice wholemeal toast with low-fat spread from
   allowance

13 5 fl oz (150 ml) unsweetened grapefruit juice
   2 oz (50 g) unsweetened muesli with skimmed milk
   from allowance

14 5 fl oz (150 ml) unsweetened orange juice
   1 boiled egg
   1 slice wholemeal toast with low-fat spread from
   allowance

SNACK MEALS

Choose one item from list A and one from list B:

Snack meal A

1 Cottage cheese and chive omelette (*see p. 251*)
  1 wholemeal roll or 2 slices wholemeal bread

2 7 oz (200 g) baked potato with Arab salad and
  cottage cheese filling (*see p. 245*)

3 Roasted pepper salad (*see p. 239*)
  1 wholemeal roll or 2 slices wholemeal bread

4 Mushrooms à la Grecque (*see p. 240*)
  1 wholemeal roll

5 Gazpacho (*see p. 231*)
  2 slices wholemeal bread

6 Carrot and dill pâté (*see p. 237*)
  2 slices wholemeal bread or toast

7 Herb and cheese-stuffed tomatoes (*see p. 247*)
  1 wholemeal roll

8 Chilled cucumber and mint soup (*see p. 230*)
  2 slices wholemeal bread

9 Greek salad (*see p. 241*)
  1 wholemeal roll

10 Quick bean soup (*see p. 235*)
  1 wholemeal roll

11 Hummus (*see p. 238*)
  1 slice wholemeal bread or 1 wholemeal pitta bread

12 Courgettes à la Grecque (*see p. 241*)
  1 wholemeal roll

13 Chilled tomato, yoghurt and basil soup (*see p. 230*)
    1 wholemeal roll

14 Cottage cheese and fruit salad (*see p. 248*)
    2 slices wholemeal bread

15 Potato and leek soup (*see p. 232*). (Use water or
    vegetable stock instead of chicken stock)

16 Tomato and red pepper soup (*see p. 234*)

17 Leeks à la Grecque (*see p. 242*)

18 Fresh mixed herb omelette (*see p. 252*)

19 Quick pea soup (*see p. 236*). (Use water or vegetable
    stock instead of chicken stock)

20 Tabbouleh (*see p. 243*)

Snack meal B

Any fruit can be accompanied by unlimited low-fat natural
yoghurt or as much 1% fromage frais as you like.

1   1 apple
2   1 pear
3   1 small banana
4   1 orange
5   2 satsumas or 2 tangerines
6   4 oz (100 g) grapes
7   4 oz (100 g) cherries
8   1 peach
9   1 nectarine
10 3 apricots
11 3 plums
12 2 fresh figs
13 Large slice melon
14 Large slice watermelon
15 Large slice fresh pineapple

16   4 oz (100 g) strawberries
17   4 oz (100 g) raspberries
18   1 diet yoghurt, any flavour
19   1 low-fat diet fromage frais, any flavour
20   4 oz (100 g) any canned fruit in natural juice.
     Choose from: apricot halves, fruit salad, grapefruit
     segments, mandarins, peaches, pears, pineapple,
     raspberries, strawberries

MAIN MEALS

*Choose any main meal from the following list, then see
p. 196 for a choice of accompaniments. Finally, choose
a pudding!*

1   Mushroom risotto (*see p. 260*)
2   Vegetable stir-fry (*see p. 266*)
3   Chick pea curry (*see p. 264*)
4   Frittata (*see p. 252*)
5   Cauliflower cheese (*see p. 264*)
6   Barbecued tofu with rice (*see p. 263*)
7   Spaghetti with mushroom sauce (*see p. 254*)
8   Vegetable chilli (*see p. 269*)
9   Broccoli risotto (*see p. 260*)
10   Mushroom, olive and caper pizza (*see p. 268*)
11   Peppers stuffed with bulgar pilaf (*see p. 270*)
12   Potato and mushroom gratin (*see p. 262*)
13   Fresh mixed herb omelette (*see p. 252*)
14   Vegetarian moussaka (*see p. 271*)
15   Spaghetti with fresh tomato and basil sauce (*see p. 256*). (Use 3–3½ oz/75–90 g of spaghetti)
16   Spaghetti with broccoli (*see p. 255*). (Use 3–3½ oz/ 75–90 g of spaghetti)
17   Cottage cheese and chive omelette (*see p. 251*)

If your main meal dish already includes rice, potatoes, pasta, noodles, bulgar wheat, or is the pizza, choose one item from list **B** and one from list **C**. (Alternatively you can pick two items from list **B** *or* two from list **C**.)

If your dish does not include rice, potatoes etc., choose one item from list **A**, one from **B** and one from **C**. (Again, you can pick two from list **B** *or* two from list **C** if you prefer.)

Main meal A
7 oz (200 g) baked potato
7 oz (200 g) boiled potatoes
Potato gratin with 7 oz
(200 g) potato (*see p. 342*)
Potato baked with lemon and
garlic with 7 oz (200 g)
potato (*see p. 343*)
2½ oz (65 g) pasta
2½ oz (65 g) noodles
2½ oz (65 g) bulgar wheat
2½ oz (65 g) brown rice

Main meal B
Up to:
3 oz (75 g) broad beans
6 oz (175 g) French beans
6 oz (175 g) Brussels sprouts
8 oz (225 g) cabbage
6 oz (175 g) broccoli
6 oz (175 g) carrots
8 oz (225 g) kale
5 oz (150 g) leeks
2 oz (50 g) parsnips
3 oz (75 g) peas
4 oz (100 g) spinach
6 oz (175 g) swede
8 oz (225 g) turnips
2 oz (50 g) sweetcorn

Or, as much as you like of the following 'free' list:

cauliflower	courgettes
celery	marrow
Chinese cabbage	mushrooms
chicory	

All vegetables to be boiled, 'dry-fried' (see p. 86), steamed or microwaved. Do not add any fat during the cooking method or while eating them.

Main meal C

Unlimited quantities except where indicated:

Tomato salad (see p. 322)
Arab salad (see p. 322)
Coleslaw (see p. 322)
Button mushroom salad (see p. 322)
Spicy tomato salad (see p. 323)
Minty cucumber salad (see p. 323)
Roasted pepper salad (see p. 239)
Pea salad with 3 oz (75 g) peas (see p. 324)
Broad bean salad with 3 oz (75 g) broad beans (see p. 324)
Mangetout salad with 3 oz (75 g) mangetout (see p. 324)
Fennel and red pepper salad (see p. 323)

Or, have limited quantities of the following 'free' list salad vegetables with, if you like, either 1 tablespoon of low-fat mayonnaise (see p. 346) or 1 quantity of any salad dressing on pp. 325–8:

alfalfa sprouts	chicory
beansprouts	lettuce (all kinds)
carrots, grated	mustard and cress
celery	peppers
Chinese leaves	radishes
cucumber	tomatoes
endive	watercress

MAIN MEAL PUDDINGS

Choose any pudding from the following:

1 *The BBC Diet* chocolate mousse (not more than once a week!) (*see p. 329*)
2 Apple cinnamon toast (*see p. 330*)
3 Strawberry mousse (*see p. 330*)
4 Oranges in orange jelly (*see p. 331*)
5 Apple jelly with grapes (*see p. 332*)
6 Fruit kebabs (*see p. 332*)
7 Baked apple with sultanas and apple juice (*see p. 334*)
8 Baked banana and orange (*see p. 335*)
9 Pear and tofu whip (*see p. 335*)
10 Banana split (*see p. 336*)
11 Strawberries with raspberry sauce (*see p. 336*)
12 Greek fruit salad (*see p. 337*)
13 Fresh fruit salad (*see p. 338*)
14 Dried fruit salad (*see p. 337*)
15 Mango cream (*see p. 338*)
16 Orange or apple blancmange (*see p. 341*)
17 Slimmers' lemon cheesecake (*see p. 340*)

THE FLEXIBLE GOURMET PLAN

(1250 calories a day)

For a more flexible version of The Gourmet Plan choose one breakfast, one snack meal and one main meal (plus pudding) for each day. You'll see that there are also guidelines for what to eat with your main meal in the way of potatoes, rice, vegetables etc. Remember, your additional allowances are as follows (sometimes mentioned in the lists but, of course, to be used as and when you like):

Daily allowance   10 fl oz (300 ml) skimmed milk
Weekly allowance 3 oz (75 g) low-fat spread

Other drinks:
Unlimited tap, still or carbonated water
Unlimited no-cal drinks
Up to 7 fl oz (200 ml) natural unsweetened fruit juice per day (in addition to any suggested in a plan)

Optional:
1 alcoholic drink per day, choosing from:
1 glass wine
½ pint beer or cider or lager
1 small sherry or port or martini
1 single measure of spirits such as whisky or gin with slimline mixer

Remember, if you don't have the alcoholic drink you'll lose weight a little more quickly.

NOTE   1 wholemeal roll should weigh about 2 oz (50 g). 1 slice of wholemeal bread should weigh about 1 oz (25 g). So, instead of 1 roll you could have 2 slices of bread (or vice versa) if you prefer.

BREAKFASTS

Choose any breakfast from:

1   5 fl oz (150 ml) unsweetened orange juice
    2 Weetabix with skimmed milk from allowance

2   4 oz (100 g) unsweetened grapefruit segments
    2 slices wholemeal toast with low-fat spread from
    allowance
    2 teaspoons reduced-sugar jam or marmalade

3   5 fl oz (150 ml) unsweetened apple juice
    1½ oz (40 g) unsweetened muesli with skimmed
    milk from allowance

4   1 oz (25 g) branflakes with skimmed milk from
    allowance
    1 slice wholemeal toast with low-fat spread from
    allowance
    1 teaspoon reduced-sugar jam or marmalade

5   5 oz (150 ml) unsweetened orange juice
    1 oz (25 g) dry oats made into porridge with water
    or skimmed milk from allowance
    1 slice wholemeal toast with low-fat spread from
    allowance
    1 teaspoon reduced-sugar jam or marmalade

6   7 oz (200 g) tin tomatoes and 1 slice wholemeal
    toast or grilled fresh tomatoes on 1 slice wholemeal
    toast

7   5 fl oz (150 ml) unsweetened orange juice
    1 boiled egg
    1 slice wholemeal bread or toast with low-fat spread
    from allowance

8 1 Shredded Wheat with skimmed milk from
   allowance
   1 slice wholemeal toast with low-fat spread from
   allowance
   1 teaspoon reduced-sugar jam or marmalade

9 5 fl oz (150 ml) unsweetened grapefruit juice
   1 oz (25 g) branflakes with skimmed milk from
   allowance

10 2 oz (50 g) unsweetened prunes
   2 slices wholemeal toast with low-fat spread from
   allowance
   2 teaspoons reduced-sugar jam or marmalade

11 4 oz (100 g) mushrooms, 'dry-fried' (see p. 86)
   1 slice wholemeal toast

12 5 fl oz (150 ml) unsweetened orange juice
   1 egg scrambled with 1 tablespoon skimmed milk
   from allowance
   1 grilled tomato
   1 slice wholemeal toast

13 5 fl oz (150 ml) unsweetened grapefruit juice
   1½ oz (40 g) unsweetened muesli with skimmed
   milk from allowance

14 5 fl oz (150 ml) unsweetened grapefruit segments
   1 boiled egg
   1 slice wholemeal bread or toast

SNACK MEALS

Choose one item from list A and one from list B:

Snack meal A

1   Avgolemono (*see p. 234*)
    1 wholemeal roll or 2 slices wholemeal bread

2   Tapénade (*see p. 237*)
    2 slices wholemeal bread or toast

3   Tomato and red pepper soup (*see p. 234*)
    1 wholemeal roll or 2 slices wholemeal bread

4   Cold trout marinated in orange (*see p. 274*)
    unlimited salad from 'free' list (*see p. 208*)
    1 wholemeal roll or 2 slices wholemeal bread

5   Salade Niçoise (*see p. 242*)
    1 wholemeal roll or 2 slices wholemeal bread

6   Tabbouleh (*see p. 243*)
    unlimited salad from 'free' list (*see p. 208*)

7   Quick gravad lax (*see p. 249*)
    unlimited salad from 'free' list (*see p. 208*)
    2 slices wholemeal bread

8   Baked potato with crispy bacon and Arab salad
    filling (*see p. 246*)

9   Tuna-stuffed pitta (*see p. 244*)

10 Gazpacho (*see p. 231*)
    1 wholemeal roll or 2 slices wholemeal bread

11 Roasted pepper salad (*see p. 239*)
    unlimited salad from 'free' list (*see p. 208*) or 1 slice
    wholemeal roll or 2 slices wholemeal bread

12 Quick bean soup (see p. 235)
    1 wholemeal roll or 2 slices wholemeal bread

13 Greek salad (see p. 241)
    1 wholemeal roll or 2 slices wholemeal bread

14 Mushrooms à la Grecque (see p. 240)
    1 wholemeal roll or 2 slices wholemeal bread

15 Cottage cheese and chive omelette (see p. 251).
    1 wholemeal roll or 2 slices wholemeal bread

16 Baked potato with Arab salad and cottage cheese
    filling (see p. 245)

17 Carrot and dill pâté (see p. 237)
    2 slices wholemeal bread or toast

18 Herb and cheese-stuffed tomatoes (see p. 247)
    1 wholemeal roll

19 Chilled cucumber and mint soup (see p. 230)
    2 slices wholemeal bread

20 Hummus (see p. 238)
    1 slice wholemeal bread, toast or 1 pitta bread

21 Courgettes à la Grecque (see p. 241)
    1 wholemeal roll

22 Chilled tomato, yoghurt and basil soup (see p. 230)
    1 wholemeal roll

23 Cottage cheese and fruit salad (see p. 248)
    2 slices wholemeal bread

24 Quick pea soup (see p. 236)
    1 wholemeal roll or 2 slices wholemeal bread

25 2 slices wholemeal bread
    2 oz (50 g) roast beef, trimmed of all fat
    cucumber or unlimited salad from the 'free' list (see
    p. 208)

26   2 oz (50 g) corned beef
    2 slices wholemeal bread
    unlimited salad from the 'free' list (*see p. 208*)

Snack meal B

Any fruit can be accompanied by unlimited low-fat natural yoghurt or as much 1% fromage frais as you like.

1   1 apple
2   1 pear
3   1 small banana
4   1 orange
5   2 satsumas or 2 tangerines
6   4 oz (100 g) grapes
7   4 oz (100 g) cherries
8   1 peach
9   1 nectarine
10   3 apricots
11   3 plums
12   2 fresh figs
13   Large slice melon
14   Large slice watermelon
15   Large slice fresh pineapple
16   4 oz (100 g) strawberries
17   4 oz (100 g) raspberries
18   1 diet yoghurt, any flavour
19   1 low-fat diet fromage frais, any flavour
20   4 oz (100 g) any tinned fruit in natural juice.
    Choose from: apricot halves, fruit salad, grapefruit segments, mandarins, peaches, pears, pineapple, raspberries, strawberries

MAIN MEALS

Choose a main meal dish and then pick the accompaniments you would like following the instructions on p. 206. Finally, choose a pudding!

1   Pork escalopes with white wine (*see p. 307*)
2   Lamb and mint kebabs with yoghurt sauce
     (*see p. 317*)
3   Stir-fried beef and broccoli (*see p. 313*)
4   Turkey 'saltimbocca' (*see p. 302*)
5   Trout with cucumber sauce (*see p. 275*)
6   Roast chicken with fresh herbs (*see p. 300*)
7   Marinated lamb cutlets (*see p. 319*)
8   Haddock with yellow pepper sauce (*see p. 277*)
9   Calf's or lamb's liver with orange and vermouth
     (*see p. 310*)
10 Turkey kebabs marinated in yoghurt, lime and
     ginger (*see p. 304*)
11 Stuffed baked trout (*see p. 273*)
12 Pasta shells with prawns, lime and dill (*see p. 289*)
13 Turkey escalopes Marsala (*see p. 303*)
14 Mushroom risotto (*see p. 260*)
15 Vegetable stir-fry (*see p. 266*)
16 Chick pea curry (*see p. 264*)
17 Frittata (*see p. 252*)
18 Cauliflower cheese (*see p. 264*)
19 Barbecued tofu with rice (*see p. 263*)
20 Spaghetti with mushroom sauce (*see p. 254*)
21 Vegetable chilli (*see p. 269*)
22 Broccoli risotto (*see p. 260*)
23 Mushroom, olive and caper pizza (*see p. 268*)
24 Peppers stuffed with bulgar pilaf (*see p. 270*)
25 Potato and mushroom gratin (*see p. 262*)
26 Fresh mixed herb omelette (*see p. 252*)

27   Vegetarian moussaka (*see p. 271*)
28   Kedgeree (*see p. 291*)
29   Spaghetti with fresh tomato and basil sauce
     (*see p. 256*)
30   Turkeyballs in mushroom and yoghurt sauce
     (*see p. 305*)
31   Grilled trout with bacon (*see p. 275*)
32   Lamb pilaf (*see p. 320*)
33   Ovenbaked crispy chicken (*see p. 296*)
34   Grilled cod with parsley sauce (*see p. 276*)
35   Tuna and mushroom supreme (*see p. 284*)
36   Chicken curry (*see p. 297*) with Fresh tomato and
     onion chutney (*see p. 344*)
37   Quick sweet and sour pork (*see p. 308*)
38   Spaghetti with broccoli (*see p. 255*)
39   Cottage cheese and chive omelette (*see p. 251*)
40   Tuna omelette (*see p. 284*)
41   Prawn and fennel risotto (*see p. 288*)
42   Grilled haddock with fromage frais (*see p. 276*)
43   Monkfish provençale (*see p. 290*)
44   Marinated and devilled chicken (*see p. 293*)

If your main meal dish already includes rice, potatoes, pasta, noodles, bulgar wheat or is the pizza, choose one item from list **B** and one from list **C**. (Alternatively you can pick two items from list **B** or two from list **C**.)

If your dish does not include rice, potatoes etc., choose one item from list **A**, one from **B** and one from **C**. (Again, you can pick two from list **B** or two from list **C** if you prefer.)

Main meal A

7 oz (200 g) baked potato
7 oz (200 g) boiled potatoes
Potato gratin with 7 oz (200 g) potato (*see p. 342*)
Potato baked with lemon and garlic with 7 oz (200 g) potato (*see p. 343*)

2½ oz (65 g) pasta
2½ oz (65 g) noodles
2½ oz (65 g) bulgar wheat
2½ oz (65 g) brown rice

Main meal B
Up to:
3 oz (75 g) broad beans
6 oz (175 g) French beans
6 oz (175 g) Brussels sprouts
8 oz (225 g) cabbage
6 oz (175 g) broccoli
6 oz (175 g) carrots
8 oz (225 g) kale
5 oz (150 g) leeks
2 oz (50 g) parsnips
3 oz (75 g) peas
4 oz (100 g) spinach
6 oz (175 g) swede
8 oz (225 g) turnips
2 oz (50 g) sweetcorn

Or, as much as you like of the following 'free' list:

cauliflower	courgettes
celery	marrow
Chinese cabbage	mushrooms
chicory	

All vegetables to be boiled, 'dry-fried' (*see p.* 86), steamed or microwaved. Do not add any fat during the cooking method or while eating them.

Main meal C

Unlimited quantities except where indicated:

Tomato salad (see p. 322)
Arab salad (see p. 322)
Coleslaw (see p. 322)
Button mushroom salad (see p. 322)
Spicy tomato salad (see p. 323)
Minty cucumber salad (see p. 323)
Roasted pepper salad (see p. 239)
Pea salad with 3 oz (75 g) peas (see p. 324)
Broad bean salad with 3 oz (75 g) broad beans (see p. 324)
Mangetout salad with 3 oz (75 g) mangetout (see p. 324)
Fennel and red pepper salad (see p. 323)

Or, have limited quantities of the following 'free' list salad vegetables with, if you like, either 1 tablespoon of low-fat mayonnaise (see p. 346) or 1 quantity of any salad dressing on pp. 325–8:

alfalfa sprouts	chicory
beansprouts	lettuce (all kinds)
carrots, grated	mustard and cress
celery	peppers
Chinese leaves	radishes
cucumber	tomatoes
endive	watercress

MAIN MEAL PUDDINGS

Choose any pudding from the following:

1   *The BBC Diet* chocolate mousse (not more than once a week!) (see p. 329)
2   Apple cinnamon toast (see p. 330)
3   Strawberry mousse (see p. 330)

THE FLEXIBLE HEARTY-EATING PLAN

(1500 calories a day)

For a more flexible plan, choose one breakfast, one snack meal and one main meal (plus pudding) for each day. You will see that there are also guidelines for what to eat with your main meal in the way of potatoes, rice, vegetables etc.

Remember, your additional allowances are as follows (sometimes mentioned in the lists but, of course, to be used as and when you like):

Daily allowance　　10 fl oz (300 ml) skimmed milk
Weekly allowance　3 oz (75 g) low-fat spread

Other drinks:
Unlimited tap, still or carbonated water
Unlimited no-cal drinks
Up to 7 fl oz (200 ml) natural unsweetened fruit juice per day (in addition to any suggested in a plan)

Optional:
1 alcoholic drink per day, choosing from:
1 glass wine
½ pint beer or cider or lager
1 small sherry or port or martini
1 single measure of spirits such as whisky or gin with slimline mixer

Remember, it's not compulsory to have the alcoholic drink! If you don't drink it, you'll lose weight a little more quickly.

NOTE　　1 wholemeal roll should weigh about 2 oz (50 g).
1 slice of wholemeal bread should weigh about 1 oz (25 g). So, instead of 1 roll you could have 2 slices of bread (or vice versa) if you prefer.

BREAKFASTS

Choose any breakfast from:

1   5 fl oz (150 ml) unsweetened orange juice
2 Weetabix with skimmed milk from allowance
1 slice wholemeal toast with low-fat spread from
allowance
1 teaspoon reduced-sugar jam or marmalade

2   5 fl oz (150 ml) unsweetened orange juice
2 rashers lean back bacon, trimmed of fat and
grilled
1 grilled tomato
2 slices wholemeal toast with low-fat spread from
allowance

3   2 rashers lean back bacon trimmed of fat and
grilled
1 small low-fat sausage, grilled
1 grilled tomato
1 slice wholemeal toast with low-fat spread from
allowance

4   2 poached eggs
2 slices wholemeal toast with low-fat spread from
allowance

5   5 fl oz (150 ml) unsweetened grapefruit juice
2 oz (50 g) dry oats made into porridge with water
or skimmed milk from allowance
1 small banana

6   5 fl oz (150 ml) unsweetened orange juice
1 boiled egg
2 slices wholemeal toast with low-fat spread from
allowance

7   5 fl oz (150 ml) unsweetened apple juice
    2 Shredded Wheat with skimmed milk from
    allowance
    1 slice wholemeal bread or toast with low-fat spread
    from allowance

8   5 fl oz (150 ml) unsweetened orange juice
    7 oz (200 g) tin tomatoes
    2 slices wholemeal toast with low-fat spread from
    allowance

9   5 fl oz (150 ml) unsweetened grapefruit juice
    1 small grilled kipper
    1 slice wholemeal toast with low-fat spread from
    allowance

10 4 oz (100 g) unsweetened grapefruit segments
    5 oz (150 g) smoked haddock fillet, poached
    1 slice wholemeal toast with low-fat spread from
    allowance

11 5 fl oz (150 ml) unsweetened orange juice
    2 Weetabix with skimmed milk from allowance
    1 slice wholemeal toast with low-fat spread from
    allowance

12 5 fl oz (150 ml) unsweetened grapefruit juice
    2 oz (50 g) dry oats made into porridge with water
    and skimmed milk from allowance
    1 small banana

SNACK MEALS

Choose one item from list A and two from list B:

Snack meal A

1   Quick pea soup (*see p. 236*)
    1 wholemeal roll or 2 slices wholemeal bread

2   Potato and leek soup (*see p. 232*)
    1 wholemeal roll or 2 slices wholemeal bread

3   Salade Niçoise (*see p. 242*)
    1 wholemeal roll or 2 slices wholemeal bread

4   Gazpacho (*see p. 231*)
    1 wholemeal roll or 2 slices wholemeal bread

5   Courgettes à la Grecque (*see p. 241*)
    2 slices wholemeal bread

6   3 slices wholemeal bread with low-fat spread from
    allowance
    3 oz (75 g) ham, trimmed of all fat
    2 tomatoes or other salad items from 'free' list on
    p. 218

7   Baked potato with crispy bacon and Arab salad
    filling (*see p. 246*)

8   Greek salad (*see p. 241*)
    2 slices wholemeal bread

9   2 slices wholemeal bread with low-fat spread from
    allowance
    2 oz (50 g) low-fat (14%) Cheddar
    2 teaspoons Branston or tomato pickle

10 Quick bean soup (*see p. 235*)
    1 wholemeal roll or 2 slices wholemeal bread

11   3 slices wholemeal bread
     3 oz (75 g) corned beef
     2 teaspoons Piccalilli

12   Hummus (*see p. 238*)
     2 slices wholemeal bread or toast

13   Tuna-stuffed potato (*see p. 246*)

14   3 slices wholemeal bread
     3 oz (75 g) roast beef, trimmed of all fat
     tomato, cucumber and lettuce or other salad items
     from 'free' list on p. 218.

In addition you can choose from the snack meals in the Vegetarian, Gourmet and No-bother flexible plans.

Snack meal B

Choose any two items from this list. Fruit can be accompanied by unlimited low-fat natural yoghurt or as much 1% fromage frais as you like.

1   1 apple
2   1 pear
3   1 small banana
4   1 orange
5   2 satsumas or 2 tangerines
6   4 oz (100 g) grapes
7   4 oz (100 g) cherries
8   1 peach
9   1 nectarine
10 3 apricots
11 3 plums
12 2 fresh figs
13 Large slice melon
14 Large slice watermelon

15 Large slice fresh pineapple
16 4 oz (100 g) strawberries
17 4 oz (100 g) raspberries
18 1 diet yoghurt, any flavour
19 1 low-fat diet fromage frais, any flavour
20 4 oz (100 g) any tinned fruit in natural juice.
    Choose from: apricot halves, fruit salad, grapefruit
    segments, mandarins, peaches, pears, pineapple,
    raspberries, strawberries

MAIN MEALS

Choose a main meal dish and then pick the accompaniments you would like following the instructions on p. 216. Finally, choose a pudding from the last list.

1   Turkey burgers (*see p. 306*)
2   Sardine fishcakes (*see p. 281*)
3   Lamb's kidneys in mushroom sauce (*see p. 318*)
4   Lamb-stuffed peppers (*see p. 321*)
5   Ovenbaked crispy chicken (*see p. 296*)
6   Steak with mustard sauce (*see p. 314*)
7   Chicken in barbecue sauce (*see p. 292*)
8   Fisherman's pie (*see p. 278*)
9   4 oz (100 g) grilled gammon, trimmed of all fat
10 Chicken stir-fry (*see p. 294*)
11 4 oz (100 g) lean leg roast lamb, trimmed of all fat
12 Mixed grill of 2 trimmed back rashers bacon (2 oz/
    50 g), 2 small low-fat sausages, 2 grilled tomatoes,
    4 oz (100 g) grilled or 'dry-fried' mushrooms
    (*see p. 86*)
13 Quick stir-fried pork with beansprouts (*see p. 308*)
14 Roast chicken with mushrooms (*see p. 298*)

You can also choose any main meal from the Vegetarian, Gourmet or No-bother flexible plans.

If your main meal dish already includes rice, potatoes, pasta, noodles, bulgar wheat or is the pizza, choose one item from list **B** and one from list **C**. (Alternatively you can pick two items from list **B** or two from list **C**.)

If your dish does not include rice, potatoes etc., choose one item from list **A**, one from **B** and one from **C**. (Again, you can pick two from list **B** or two from list **C** if you prefer.)

Main meal A
7–9 oz (200–250 g) baked potato
7–9 oz (200–250 g) boiled potatoes
Potato gratin with 7–9 oz
(200–250 g) potatoes
(see p. 342)
Potato baked with lemon and
garlic with 7–9 oz (200–250 g)
potatoes (see p. 343)
3 oz (75 g) pasta
3 oz (75 g) noodles
3 oz (75 g) bulgar wheat
3 oz (75 g) brown rice

Main meal B
Up to:
3 oz (75 g) broad beans
6 oz (175 g) French beans
6 oz (175 g) Brussels sprouts
8 oz (225 g) cabbage
6 oz (175 g) broccoli
6 oz (175 g) carrots
8 oz (225 g) kale
5 oz (150 g) leeks
2 oz (50 g) parsnips

3 oz (75 g) peas
4 oz (100 g) spinach
6 oz (175 g) swede
8 oz (225 g) turnips
2 oz (50 g) sweetcorn

Or, as much as you like of the following 'free' list:

cauliflower	courgettes
celery	marrow
Chinese cabbage	mushrooms
chicory	

All vegetables to be boiled, 'dry-fried' (see p. 86), steamed or microwaved. Do not add any fat during the cooking method or while eating them.

Main meal C

Unlimited quantities except where indicated:

Tomato salad (see p. 322)
Arab salad (see p. 322)
Coleslaw (see p. 322)
Button mushroom salad (see p. 322)
Spicy tomato salad (see p. 323)
Minty cucumber salad (see p. 323)
Roasted pepper salad (see p. 239)
Pea salad with 3 oz (75 g) peas (see p. 324)
Broad bean salad with 3 oz (75 g) broad beans (see p. 324)
Mangetout salad with 3 oz (75 g) mangetout (see p. 324)
Fennel and red pepper salad (see p. 323)

Or, have limited quantities of the following 'free' list salad vegetables with, if you like, either 1 tablespoon of low-fat mayonnaise (see p. 346) or 1 quantity of any salad dressing on pp. 325–8:

alfalfa sprouts

beansprouts

carrots, grated

celery

Chinese leaves

cucumber

endive

chicory

mustard and cress

peppers

radishes

tomatoes

watercress

MAIN MEAL PUDDINGS

Choose any pudding from:

1 *The BBC Diet* chocolate mousse (not more than once a week!) (*see p. 329*)
2 Apple cinnamon toast (*see p. 330*)
3 Strawberry mousse (*see p. 330*)
4 Oranges in orange jelly (*see p. 331*)
5 Apple jelly with grapes (*see p. 332*)
6 Fruit kebabs (*see p. 332*)
7 Baked apple with sultanas and apple juice (*see p. 334*)
8 Baked banana and orange (*see p. 335*)
9 Pear and tofu whip (*see p. 335*)
10 Banana split (*see p. 336*)
11 Strawberries with raspberry sauce (*see p. 336*)
12 Greek fruit salad (*see p. 337*)
13 Fresh fruit salad (*see p. 338*)
14 Dried fruit salad (*see p. 337*)
15 Mango cream (*see p. 338*)
16 Orange or apple blancmange (*see p. 341*)
17 Slimmers' lemon cheesecake (*see p. 340*)

THE NO-BOTHER PLAN

(1250 calories a day)

This is a 'middle way' flexible plan using convenience foods or very easy to prepare 'no recipe' meals. It's satisfactory for most women unless they're of below average height or very inactive. If you are such a woman you could use this plan and increase your physical activity. Nearly all men will lose weight quickly on this plan.

To follow The No-bother Plan you need to choose one breakfast, one snack meal and one main meal (plus a pudding) for each day.

The additional allowances are as follows (these are sometimes mentioned in the plans but, of course, you may use them as and when you like):

Daily allowance   10 fl oz (300 ml) skimmed milk
Weekly allowance   3 oz (75 g) low-fat spread

Other drinks:
Unlimited tap, still or carbonated water
Unlimited no-cal drinks
Up to 7 fl oz (200 ml) natural unsweetened fruit juice per day (in addition to any suggested in a plan)

Optional:
1 alcoholic drink per day, choosing from:
1 glass wine
½ pint beer or cider or lager
1 small sherry or port or martini
1 single measure of spirits such as whisky or gin with slimline mixer

Remember, if you don't have the alcoholic drink you'll lose weight a little more quickly.

NOTE   1 wholemeal roll should weigh about 2 oz (50 g).
1 slice of wholemeal bread should weigh about
1 oz (25 g).

So, instead of 1 roll you could have 2 slices of
bread (or vice versa) if you prefer.

BREAKFASTS

*Choose any breakfast from the Quickfire, Vegetarian
or Gourmet Plans (see pp. 181, 191 and 200). You
can pick a different one for each day or have the same
one every day – it's up to you.*

SNACK MEALS

Choose one item from list A and one from list B:

Snack meal A

1   1 × 7 oz (200 g) tin reduced-sugar baked beans
    2 slices wholemeal toast

2   7 oz (200 g) baked potato
    1 × 7 oz (200 g) tin reduced-sugar baked beans

3   1 × 7 oz (200 g) tin spaghetti
    2 slices wholemeal toast

4   scrambled eggs (2 eggs cooked in non-stick pan
    using 2 tablespoons skimmed milk from allowance)
    2 slices wholemeal toast

5   2 poached eggs
    2 slices wholemeal toast

6   2 boiled eggs
    2 slices wholemeal toast or bread

7   omelette (use 2 eggs and a non-stick pan)
    choose a filling from: fresh herbs, tomatoes or 'dry-
    fried' mushrooms (*see p. 86*)
    2 slices wholemeal bread or 1 wholemeal roll

8   2 oz (50 g) (14%) Cheddar cheese
    2 slices wholemeal toast

9   1 tin sardines in brine, drained
    2 slices wholemeal toast

10 1 × 7 oz (200 g) tin ravioli
    2 slices wholemeal toast

11 1 × 7 oz (200 g) tin sausage and beans
    1 slice wholemeal toast

12 10 fl oz (300 ml) tinned vegetable (not cream) or
    packet soup with 1 wholemeal roll or 2 slices
    wholemeal bread

13 5 pieces of any fruit (but not more than 1 banana)

14 2 diet yoghurts and 2 pieces of fruit (but not more
    than 1 banana)

15 2 oz (50 g) low-fat burger, grilled
    1 wholemeal bun
    unlimited salad from 'free' list on p. 218

16 1 sandwich made from 2 slices wholemeal bread or
    1 wholemeal roll and 2 oz (50 g) ham, trimmed of
    all fat
    or 2 oz (50 g) corned beef
    or 2 oz (50 g) grated (14%) Cheddar cheese and 1
    tablespoon pickle
    or 2 oz (50 g) roast beef, trimmed of all fat
    or 3 oz (75 g) skinless, cooked chicken breast

or ½ tin (60 g) sardines in brine, drained
or 3 oz (75 g) tuna in brine or water, drained
and unlimited salad from 'free' list on p. 218

17   2 large fresh tomatoes, grilled in slices (add fresh
     herbs or garlic if you like)
     2 slices wholemeal toast or 1 × 7 oz (200 g) tin
     tomatoes
     2 slices wholemeal toast

18   4–8 oz (100–225 g) 'dry-fried' mushrooms (*see p. 86*)
     2 slices wholemeal toast

19   Ham salad with 2 oz (50 g) ham, trimmed of all fat
     any salad from 'free' list on p.218
     2 slices wholemeal bread

20   Beef salad with 2 oz (50 g) lean beef, trimmed of all
     fat
     any salad from 'free' list on p. 218
     2 slices wholemeal bread

21   Corned beef salad with 2 oz (50 g) corned beef
     any salad from 'free' list on p. 218
     2 slices wholemeal bread

22   Prawn salad with 4 oz (100 g) prawns
     any salad from 'free' list on p. 218
     2 slices wholemeal bread

23   Crab salad with 3 oz (75 g) crab (fresh, frozen or
     tinned)
     any salad from 'free' list on p. 218
     2 slices wholemeal bread

24   Salmon salad with 3 oz (75 g) tinned salmon
     any salad from 'free' list on p. 218
     2 slices wholemeal bread

25 Chicken salad with 3 oz (75 g) cooked chicken
    breast, skin removed
    any salad from 'free' list on p. 218
    2 slices wholemeal bread

Snack meal B

Choose any two items from this list. Fruit can be accompanied by unlimited low-fat natural yoghurt or as much 1% fromage frais as you like.

    1   1 apple
    2   1 pear
    3   1 small banana
    4   1 orange
    5   2 satsumas or 2 tangerines
    6   4 oz (100 g) grapes
    7   4 oz (100 g) cherries
    8   1 peach
    9   1 nectarine
    10 3 apricots
    11 3 plums
    12 2 fresh figs
    13 Large slice melon
    14 Large slice watermelon
    15 Large slice fresh pineapple
    16 4 oz (100 g) strawberries
    17 4 oz (100 g) raspberries
    18 1 diet yoghurt, any flavour
    19 1 low-fat diet fromage frais, any flavour
    20 4 oz (100 g) any tinned fruit in natural juice.
        Choose from: apricot halves, fruit salad, grapefruit
        segments, mandarins, peaches, pears, pineapple,
        raspberries, strawberries

MAIN MEALS

Choose any main meal from the following:

1   4 oz (100 g) oven chips (*see p. 228*)
    1 × 7 oz (200 g) tin reduced-sugar baked beans
    1 poached egg

2   4 oz (100 g) oven chips (*see p. 228*)
    1 poached egg
    2 small low-fat sausages, grilled

3   1 × 7 oz (200 g) baked potato
    2 small low-fat sausages, grilled
    1 × 7 oz (200 g) tin reduced-sugar baked beans

4   4 oz (100 g) oven chips (*see p. 227*)
    2 oz (50 g) low-fat burger, grilled
    2 large tomatoes, grilled
    3 oz (75 g) peas

5   4 oz (100 g) gammon steak, trimmed of all fat and
    grilled
    2 large tomatoes, grilled
    1 × 7 oz (200 g) baked potato

6   3 oz (75 g) loin lamb chop, trimmed of all fat and
    grilled
    1 teaspoon mint sauce
    5–7 oz (150–200 g) boiled potatoes
    any vegetable from 'free' list on p. 217

7   3 oz (75 g) rump steak, trimmed of all fat and
    grilled
    4 oz (100 g) oven chips (*see p. 228*)
    3 oz (75 g) peas
    2 large tomatoes, grilled

8   3 oz (75 g) pork loin chop, trimmed of all fat and grilled
1 × 7 oz (200 g) baked potato
2 oz (50 g) sweetcorn or a portion of any vegetable from 'free' list on p. 217

9   2 large low-fat sausages, grilled
5–7 oz (150–200 g) potatoes, boiled and mashed with 2 tablespoons of skimmed milk
a portion of any vegetable from 'free' list on p. 217

10   any frozen slimmers' meal of 300–350 calories

11   5 oz (150 g) grilled *or* poached fish (cod *or* haddock)
5–7 oz (150–200 g) boiled potatoes
3 oz (75 g) peas
2 large tomatoes, grilled

12   2 fish fingers, grilled
4 oz (100 g) oven chips (*see p.* 228)
3 oz (75 g) peas
2 large tomatoes, grilled

13   4 oz (100 g) bought roast chicken breast, skin removed
unlimited salad from the 'free' list on p. 218
1 × 7 oz (200 g) baked potato

14   3 oz (75 g) ham, trimmed of all fat
any salad from 'free' list on p. 218
1 × 7 oz (200 g) baked potato

15   2 hard-boiled eggs
any salad from 'free' list on p. 218
1 × 7 oz (200 g) baked potato

16   2½ oz (65 g) half-fat (14%) Cheddar cheese
any salad from 'free' list on p. 218
1 × 7 oz (200 g) baked potato

17   14 oz (400 g) reduced-sugar baked beans
      2 slices wholemeal toast

18   1 × 6 oz (175 g) trout, grilled
      5–7 oz (150–200 g) potatoes, boiled
      6 oz (175 g) broccoli or salad from 'free' list on
      p. 218

19   1 × 7 oz (200 g) tin spaghetti
      1 poached egg
      2 slices wholemeal toast

20   3 oz (75 g) roast beef, trimmed of all fat
      3 slices wholemeal bread
      any salad from 'free' list on p. 218

21   4 oz (100 g) smoked mackerel
      2 slices wholemeal bread
      any salad from 'free' list on p. 218

22   4 oz (100 g) smoked mackerel or kipper, served hot
      5–7 oz (150–200 g) potatoes, boiled
      6 oz (175 g) broccoli or any other vegetable from
      'free' list on p. 217

23   2 oz (50 g) back bacon, all fat removed, grilled
      or 1 slice back bacon and 1 small low-fat sausage,
      grilled
      2 tomatoes, grilled
      4 oz (100 g) mushrooms, 'dry-fried' (see p. 86) or
      grilled
      1 poached egg
      1 slice wholemeal bread or toast

24   3 oz (75 g) tuna in brine or water, drained
      any salad from 'free' list on p. 218
      3 slices wholemeal bread

25 4 oz (100 g) prawns
any salad from 'free' list on p. 218
3 slices wholemeal bread

26 4 oz (100 g) (including skin and bone) fresh salmon,
poached
any salad from 'free' list on p. 218
3 slices wholemeal bread

27 3 oz (75 g) tinned salmon
any salad from 'free' list on p. 218
3 slices wholemeal bread

28 4 oz (100 g) lamb's liver, 'dry-fried' (see p. 86) or
grilled
4 oz (100 g) onions, 'dry-fried' (see p. 86)
5–7 oz (150–200 g) potatoes, boiled
any vegetable from the 'free' list on p. 217

29 4 oz (100 g) crab (fresh, frozen or tinned)
any salad from 'free' list on p. 218
3 slices wholemeal bread

30 3 oz (75 g) lean roast lamb, trimmed of all fat
5–7 oz (150–200 g) potatoes, boiled or steamed
any 2 vegetables from the 'free' list on p. 217
2 tablespoons gravy
1 teaspoon mint sauce

31 3 oz (75 g) lean roast beef, trimmed of all fat
5–7 oz (150–200 g) potatoes, boiled or steamed
any 2 vegetables from the 'free' list on p. 217
2 tablespoons gravy
1 teaspoon horseradish *or* mustard

32 4 oz (100 g) lean roast chicken *or* turkey breast, skin
    removed
    5 oz (150 g) potatoes, boiled
    any 2 vegetables from the 'free' list on p. 217
    2 tablespoons gravy
    1 teaspoon stuffing

You may be surprised to see oven chips here but they are lower in calories than ones you would make yourself. However, they are still not low-calorie food and you must be careful to weigh them out accurately. Cook them in the oven or grill them and then drain well on kitchen paper before you eat them. Also, for your health's sake, try to choose a brand which uses sunflower oil.

MAIN MEAL PUDDINGS

Choose any pudding from:

1 1 diet yoghurt, fruit-flavoured
2 2 oz (50 g) vanilla ice-cream
3 2 oz (50 g) vanilla ice-cream with 1 piece fresh fruit
4 2 pieces fresh fruit
5 1 piece fresh fruit and 1 diet yoghurt
6 2 diet yoghurts
7 2 low-fat slimmers' fromage frais
8 unlimited low-fat natural yoghurt or as much 1% fromage frais as you like with 4 oz (100 g) any tinned fruit in natural juice. Choose from: apricot halves, fruit salad, grapefruit segments, mandarins, peaches, pears, pineapple, raspberries, strawberries

19 The Recipes

In all the recipes the spoon measurements are level ones unless it says otherwise. I have taken as a teaspoon measure a 5 ml spoon and a 15 ml spoon for a tablespoon.

Metric conversions are given for all quantities and remember to use *either* the imperial *or* metric measurements consistently throughout a recipe.

SOUPS

CHILLED CUCUMBER AND MINT SOUP

SERVES 2
½ large cucumber
10 oz (275 g) low-fat natural yoghurt
5 fl oz (150 ml) cold Chicken stock (see p. 348) or
5 fl oz (150 ml) skimmed milk
1–2 cloves garlic, peeled
6–8 leaves fresh mint
salt and freshly milled black pepper

* Reserve a 2–3 inch (5–7.5 cm) piece of cucumber and put the rest in a liquidiser or food processor with the yoghurt, stock or milk, garlic and mint. Process until smooth.
* Finely dice the remaining cucumber and fold it into the soup.
* Chill for at least 2 hours. Season to taste before serving.

CHILLED TOMATO, YOGHURT AND BASIL SOUP

This is a beautiful pink and green-flecked summer soup with the haunting taste of fresh basil. It's very easy to make but don't be tempted to use dried basil: it just doesn't taste the same. If you can't get hold of fresh basil, use another fresh herb like chives, parsley or about 1 tablespoon of mint.

SERVES 2
1 × 14-oz (400-g) tin tomatoes
5 oz (150 g) low-fat natural yoghurt
2 tablespoons chopped, fresh basil
salt and freshly milled black pepper
basil leaves to garnish (optional)

❋ Put the tomatoes, yoghurt and basil in a liquidiser or food processor and process for 1–2 minutes or until smooth.

❋ Chill the soup for at least 2 hours. Season to taste.

❋ Serve in chilled soup bowls with a pair of basil leaves floating on top if you like.

GAZPACHO

This is a lovely Spanish soup which is filling – a salad in a soup bowl! A mixture of red and green pepper is nicest but, if you prefer, you could use a whole one of either instead.

SERVES 2
2–3 inch (5–7.5 cm) piece of cucumber
½ small red pepper and ½ small green pepper
1-pint (600-ml) tin tomato juice or
1 × 14-oz (400-g) tin tomatoes and 5 fl oz (150 ml) water
½ small onion or 4 spring onions
1–2 cloves garlic, peeled
1 tablespoon wine vinegar or juice of ½ lemon (to taste)
salt and freshly milled black pepper

❋ Reserve about a third of the cucumber and the peppers and chop them into ¼-inch (5-mm) cubes.

❋ Put the rest of the cucumber and peppers along with the tomato juice, or tomatoes and water, onion, garlic and wine vinegar or lemon juice into a liquidiser or food processor.

❋ Process for 1–2 minutes until smooth.
Chill the soup and the cucumber and pepper dice separately for at least 2 hours. Then taste and season the soup.

❋ Serve in chilled soup bowls, either mixing the diced cucumber and peppers into the soup just before serving, or handing them round separately to be mixed in at the table.

POTATO AND LEEK SOUP

This has a wholesome flavour and is quite filling.

SERVES 2

8 oz (225 g) leeks
4 oz (100 g) potatoes
1 pint (600 ml) Chicken stock (see p. 348) or water
salt and freshly milled black pepper
2 tablespoons 8% fromage frais or Greek yoghurt (see p. 90)
chopped fresh parsley to garnish (optional)

❋ Use the white of the leeks and 3 or 4 inches (7.5 or 10 cm)
of the green also. Wash them well, cutting them lengthways
and washing out any grit. Then cut into thick slices.
❋ Peel the potato or potatoes and cut into fine dice.
❋ Simmer the potatoes and leeks in the stock or water for
20–25 minutes until very soft.
❋ Liquidise the vegetables and their cooking liquid in a
liquidiser or food processor until smooth.
❋ Re-heat gently and season according to taste.
❋ When the soup is at boiling point, take it off the heat and
whisk in the fromage frais or Greek yoghurt.
❋ Serve immediately, sprinkling with a little chopped parsley
if you like.

LEEK AND CARROT SOUP

SERVES 4

2½ pints (1.5 litre) Chicken stock (see p. 348)
1 lb (450 g) trimmed leeks, washed thoroughly and chopped
8 oz (225 g) carrots, peeled and chopped
pinch of ground nutmeg (optional)
salt and freshly milled black pepper

❋ Place the stock, vegetables and nutmeg in a pan, bring to the boil and simmer until the vegetables are tender.
❋ Liquidise the vegetables and stock in a liquidiser or food processor until smooth.
❋ Season to taste and serve.

GARDEN VEGETABLE SOUP

SERVES 4
3 oz (75 g) green beans
2 sticks celery
2 medium potatoes, peeled
2 medium carrots, peeled
½ green pepper, de-seeded
1 medium courgette
salt and freshly milled black pepper
16 fl oz (475 ml) tomato juice or 1 × 14-oz (400-g) tin tomatoes
1 pint (600 ml) beef or Chicken stock (see p. 348)

❋ Dice all of the vegetables.
❋ Add the vegetables and seasoning to taste to the tomato juice or tinned tomatoes and stock.
❋ Bring to the boil and simmer until the vegetables are cooked.
❋ Serve hot.

TOMATO AND RED PEPPER SOUP

A warming and satisfying soup which can be made spicy if you prefer by adding the Tabasco sauce.

SERVES 2
1 red pepper, de-seeded and diced
1 small or ½ large onion, diced
1–2 cloves garlic, peeled and finely diced
1 × 14-oz (400-g) tin tomatoes
2–3 drops Tabasco sauce (optional)
salt and freshly milled black pepper

❋ 'Dry-fry' the red pepper, onion and garlic (see p. 86) in a heavy non-stick frying-pan for 7–8 minutes.
❋ Put the tomatoes and the contents of the frying-pan (adding a little water to it and stirring vigorously to dislodge any pieces that stick to the bottom) into a liquidiser or food processor. Process for 1–2 minutes or until smooth.
❋ Pour the soup into a pan and simmer gently for 5 minutes.
❋ Add Tabasco (if using) and season to taste.
❋ Serve in warmed soup bowls.

AVGOLEMONO

This Greek soup is delicious and refreshing.

SERVES 2
2 level tablespoons brown rice
1 pint (600 ml) Chicken stock (see p. 348)
1 egg
juice of ½–1 lemon
salt and freshly milled black pepper
chopped fresh parsley to garnish (optional)

* Gently simmer the rice in the Chicken stock for 30–35 minutes or until soft.
* Whisk the egg and ½ the lemon juice together in a bowl until light and fluffy.
* Pour the boiling stock and rice onto the egg and lemon mixture and return the soup to the pan. Heat gently for 1–2 minutes until very hot, but DO NOT BOIL. Season to taste and add more lemon juice if needed.
* Serve in warmed soup bowls and sprinkle with chopped parsley if you like.

QUICK BEAN SOUP

Here's a hearty filling soup, which you may find too much for one (isn't that a luxury on a diet?!). If so, keep half until the next day or freeze it.

SERVES 1

1 × 14-oz (400-g) tin cannellini (white kidney) beans
1 clove garlic, peeled
salt and freshly milled black pepper
squeeze of lemon juice
1 tablespoon finely chopped fresh parsley

* Drain the beans, reserving ½ cup of their juice. Make this up to a whole cup with water.
* Put half the beans, the diluted bean juice and the garlic into a liquidiser or food processor and process until smooth.
* Turn out into a pan and add the reserved beans. Heat gently and simmer for a couple of minutes. Add a little more water if the soup is too thick.
* Season with salt, freshly milled black pepper and lemon juice to taste. Stir in the chopped parsley just before serving.

QUICK PEA SOUP
....

Here's a soup which is as quick as a packet or tin and ten times as good.

SERVES 1
4 oz (100 g) frozen peas
10 fl oz (300 ml) Chicken stock (see p. 348)
½–1 tablespoon chopped fresh mint (optional)
1 tablespoon 8% fromage frais or Greek yoghurt (see p. 90)
salt and freshly milled black pepper

* Simmer the peas in stock for 2–3 minutes or until they are cooked. Add the mint if using.
* Liquidise or process the soup with the fromage frais or yoghurt. Re-heat gently if you need to but do not boil.
* Season to taste.

STARTERS AND SNACKS

CARROT AND DILL PÂTÉ

Serve this soft pâté with wholemeal Melba toast or crisp pitta bread (see p. 88).

SERVES 2
8 oz (225 g) carrots
2 tablespoons low-fat natural yoghurt
1 tablespoon finely chopped fresh dill
salt and freshly milled black pepper
juice of ½ lemon

✱ Scrub or peel the carrots and cut them into thick slices. Simmer in slightly salted water for 10–15 minutes or until just tender but still firm. Drain and leave until cold.

✱ Put the carrots in a liquidiser or food processor along with the yoghurt and dill and process for 1–2 minutes until smooth.

✱ Season and add lemon juice to taste.

TAPÉNADE

This is a dark, rich-tasting spread from Provence (tapéno is the Provençal dialect word for capers). Traditionally it's packed with olive oil (and therefore calories!) but this low-calorie version is very tasty. Serve with wholemeal Melba toast or crisp pitta bread (see p. 88). It is possible to buy cans of ready-stoned black olives, or you can, of course, stone your own.

SERVES 2

3 oz (75 g) stoned black olives in brine, drained on kitchen paper
1 oz (25 g) anchovy fillets, very well drained
2 oz (50 g) tuna in brine or water, drained
1–2 tablespoons capers, drained
3–4 tablespoons tomato juice or 3–4 teaspoons tomato purée mixed
with 3–4 tablespoons water
1 tablespoon wine vinegar or juice of ½ lemon

✳ Put everything, except the wine vinegar or lemon juice, into
a liquidiser or food processor and process for a minute or
so or until you have a smooth dark paste.

✳ Add the wine vinegar or lemon juice to taste, adding more
if needed.

✳ Serve cold with the hot Melba toast or pitta bread.

HUMMUS

*This moreish Greek spread is normally laden with olive oil, but this
low-calorie version is just as good. Serve with wholemeal Melba toast
or crisp pitta bread (see p. 88) or simply warmed wholemeal pitta
bread.*

SERVES 2

3½ oz (90 g) dried chick peas or 1 × 14-oz (400-g) tin chick peas
2 cloves garlic, peeled
3 tablespoons low-fat natural yoghurt
juice of ½–1 lemon
salt and freshly milled black pepper
2 tablespoons chopped fresh parsley or ½ teaspoon paprika

✳ If using dried chick peas, soak them in water overnight:
throw away the soaking water; bring to the boil and simmer
them in fresh water until tender. This may take an hour or
more depending on the vintage of your chick peas!

✳ Put the cold, drained chick peas, or the drained tinned chick peas into a liquidiser or food processor along with the garlic, yoghurt and lemon juice and process until smooth. Season to taste.

✳ Serve on a flat dish decorated with the parsley or sprinkled with the paprika.

ROASTED PEPPER SALAD

It sounds a little fiddly – though it's really quite simple – but charring peppers in this way gives them a splendid smoky flavour and the texture is quite different from fresh peppers too.

SERVES 1

2 peppers – red, yellow or green or a mixture
1 tablespoon chopped fresh parsley
1 clove garlic, peeled and finely chopped (optional)
juice of ½ lemon
salt and freshly milled black pepper

✳ Char the peppers either by cutting them in half lengthwise and placing them under a hot grill. Alternatively, place them, whole, directly on the grid of a gas hob and turn them constantly for 5–7 minutes with a pair of tongs. They need to be blistered and black all over. Leave them to cool.

✳ Peel the cooled peppers under a running cold tap. The skin comes off very easily. Remove all the black skin. Then core them and remove the seeds and any white pith.

✳ Slice the peppers into ½-inch (1-cm) strips. Sprinkle them with the parsley and finely chopped garlic (if using), spoon over the lemon juice, and season with salt and freshly ground black pepper.

✳ Leave them in a cool place for an hour or so for the flavours to blend but don't refrigerate.

MUSHROOMS À LA GRECQUE

In spite of its name, this is a French way of serving cooked vegetables cold and is usually swimming in olive oil. This version is very refreshing and just as tasty. Instead of mushrooms you could use courgettes or leeks as the variations show.

SERVES 1

1 large or 2 medium tomatoes, finely chopped (skinned if preferred)
2 tablespoons dry white wine or dry vermouth or water
2 tablespoons orange juice
1–2 teaspoons white wine vinegar or cider vinegar
1–2 cloves garlic, peeled and halved
6–10 coriander seeds, crushed
a couple of sprigs fresh parsley
a sprig of fresh thyme or small pinch of dried
½ dried bay leaf (optional)
4–6 oz (100–175) button mushrooms, wiped and left whole
salt and freshly milled black pepper
squeeze of lemon (optional)
chopped fresh parsley to garnish

* Put the tomatoes, wine or water, orange juice, vinegar, garlic, coriander and herbs in a small pan. Bring to the boil and simmer for 2–3 minutes.
* Add the mushrooms and simmer for a further 3–4 minutes until the mushrooms are soft and the liquid is reduced by about half its original volume.
* Leave to cool and remove the garlic and herb sprigs. Serve at room temperature, having seasoned to taste with salt freshly milled black pepper, and lemon juice. Sprinkle with the chopped parsley.

COURGETTES À LA GRECQUE

✳ Follow the recipe for Mushrooms à la Grecque using 4–6 oz (100–175 g) of thickly sliced courgettes in place of the mushrooms.

LEEKS À LA GRECQUE

✳ Follow the recipe for Mushrooms à la Grecque using 4–6 oz (100–175 g) of well-washed and thickly sliced leeks in place of the mushrooms.

GREEK SALAD

This is a lovely combination of tastes and takes seconds to prepare.

SERVES 1
2 tomatoes
3–4 inch (7.5–10 cm) piece cucumber (peeled if you wish)
8 black olives, unstoned
1½ oz (40 g) Feta cheese, cubed
3–4 spring onions, chopped or 1 tablespoon finely chopped onion
1 tablespoon fresh oregano, mint or parsley or a mixture, finely chopped
juice of ½ lemon
salt and freshly milled black pepper
lettuce to garnish (optional)

✳ Quarter the tomatoes and cut the cucumber into chunks. Mix them with the olives, cheese, onion and herbs. Stir in the lemon juice and season to taste. Leave for ½–1 hour for the juices to flow and flavours to mingle.
✳ Serve on its own or on a bed of lettuce.

SALADE NIÇOISE
....

This salad from the Queen of the Riviera, Nice, has as many 'authentic' recipes as there are Niçois! Here's an unauthentic but very tasty one.

SERVES 1
2 tomatoes
3-inch (7.5-cm) piece cucumber
juice of ½ lemon
salt and freshly milled black pepper
crisp lettuce leaves like Cos or Little Gem (as many as you want!)
3–4 anchovy fillets
2 oz (50 g) tuna in brine or water
6–8 black olives, unstoned
finely chopped fresh parsley to garnish

❋ Quarter the tomatoes and cut the cucumber into chunks. Pour over the lemon juice with some salt and pepper. Leave for a few minutes until the juices start to flow. These are going to be your dressing.

❋ Arrange the lettuce leaves on a plate or in a small bowl. Arrange the tomatoes and cucumber on top and sprinkle with all the juice that came out of them.

❋ Drain the anchovy fillets – best done on kitchen paper – and the tuna. Then arrange attractively on top of the salad with the black olives. Sprinkle with parsley.

NOTE If you have any handy, you could add some cooked cold French beans or some slices of red pepper to this dish. The extra calories are insignificant.

TABBOULEH
....

This traditional Lebanese salad usually comes loaded with calories in the form of olive oil, but guess what? Yep! – but it still tastes pretty good.

SERVES 1

1½ oz (40 g) bulgar wheat (burghul, pourgouri, or cracked wheat)
4–6 spring onions, finely chopped
1–2 tablespoons finely chopped fresh parsley
1 tablespoon finely chopped fresh mint
3-inch (7.5-cm) piece cucumber, finely chopped
1–2 tomatoes, finely chopped
juice of ½–1 lemon
salt and freshly milled black pepper
Little Gem or Cos lettuce leaves to serve

❋ Pour cold water over the bulgar wheat and leave it to soak for 15–20 minutes. (It's already cooked and this process makes it swell.) Drain it in a fine sieve and then take handfuls of it and squeeze as much water out as you can. Place in a bowl.

❋ Stir in the chopped onions, parsley, mint, cucumber, and tomatoes. Then mix in the lemon juice, salt and freshly milled black pepper until it tastes as you would like it.
If possible, leave to stand for a little while to allow the flavours to blend. This isn't essential, though. Serve with Little Gem or Cos lettuce leaves to scoop it up with.

TUNA-STUFFED PITTA

....

SERVES 1

2 oz (50 g) button mushrooms, wiped
1 tablespoon low-fat natural yoghurt
1 tablespoon chopped fresh parsley or chives
salt and freshly milled black pepper
squeeze of lemon juice
2 oz (50 g) tuna in brine or water, drained and flaked
1 large wholemeal pitta bread, halved

✳ Slice the mushrooms finely and add them to the yoghurt with the parsley (or chives). Stir well. Season with salt and freshly milled black pepper and lemon juice. Stir in the tuna and then warm the pitta bread halves and stuff them with the mixture.

NOTE You could also stuff the pitta bread with the tuna mixture described on p. 246.

TUNA POT RICE

....

SERVES 1

4 oz (100 g) cooked brown rice
1 oz (25 g) cooked peas or diced cucumber
1 oz (25 g) sweetcorn or chopped celery
2 oz (50 g) tuna fish in brine or water, drained and flaked
¼ green pepper, de-seeded and chopped
1 tablespoon chopped onion or three spring onions, chopped
squeeze of lemon juice
salt and freshly milled black pepper
1 tablespoon chopped fresh parsley or other herbs

✳ Mix all the ingredients together. Serve cold.

BAKED POTATO WITH ARAB SALAD AND COTTAGE CHEESE FILLING

This is a really enjoyable, virtually fat-free filling for a baked potato. Check the instructions in the diet plan you are following to see what size potato to use. The finely diced vegetables somehow add up to more than the sum of the parts. This is also good stuffed into hot wholemeal pitta bread.

SERVES 1

1 × 5-7 oz (150-200 g) potato
2 tomatoes
3-inch (7.5-cm) piece cucumber
2 or 3 spring onions or 2 teaspoons finely chopped onion
juice of ½ a small lemon
salt and freshly milled black pepper
3 tablespoons cottage cheese

✳ Clean the potato and pierce it a couple of times with a knife. Bake in a moderate oven (gas mark 4, 350°F, 180°C) for 1–1½ hours until soft. Alternatively, microwave it according to your instruction book.

✳ Meanwhile, dice the tomatoes and cucumber into pieces about as small as the nail of your little finger. Mix with the chopped onion, lemon juice and seasoning and let the mixture stand while the potato is cooking.

✳ Halve the potato and score the flesh several times with a knife to enable the juices from the vegetables to penetrate.

✳ Mix the cottage cheese and salad. Stuff the potato halves.

BAKED POTATO WITH CRISPY BACON AND ARAB SALAD FILLING

....

You could also use this tasty mixture as a stuffing for a warm piece of pitta bread. Check the instructions in the diet plan you are following to see what size potato you should use here.

SERVES 1

1 × 5-9 oz (150-250 g) potato
1½–2 oz (40–50 g) back rashers bacon, smoked or unsmoked
2 tomatoes
3-inch (7.5-cm) piece cucumber
2–3 spring onions or 2 teaspoons finely chopped onion
juice of ½ a small lemon
salt and freshly milled black pepper

* Clean the potato and pierce a couple of times with a knife. Bake in the oven at gas mark 4, 350°F (180°C) for 1–1½ hours or until cooked. Alternatively, microwave it according to your instruction book.
* Trim all the fat from the bacon and cut into small dice. 'Dry-fry' (see p. 86) until crispy. Get rid of any fat by draining the bacon pieces on some kitchen paper.
* Dice the tomatoes and cucumber into pieces the size of your little fingernail. Stir in the chopped onion, lemon juice and seasoning. Let it all stand while the potato cooks.
* Halve the cooked potato and score the flesh several times with a knife so the juices from the vegetables penetrate.
* Mix the bacon, warm or cold as wished, with the salad and stuff into the potato halves.

NOTE An alternative filling can be made using 2 oz (50 g) tinned tuna, sardines or mackerel instead of the bacon. Use fish that has been tinned in brine or water and drain well before using.

HERB AND CHEESE-STUFFED TOMATOES

Here's a quick and satisfying lunch idea. It's as easy as a sandwich but somehow, perhaps because you use a knife and fork, it seems more substantial.

SERVES 1

1 large beef tomato or *2 large ordinary tomatoes*
4 tablespoons cottage cheese
1 tablespoon 8% fromage frais (see p. 90)
1 tablespoon finely chopped fresh herbs (basil, parsley, chives, tarragon, mint or *dill* or *a combination)*
salt and freshly milled black pepper
squeeze of lemon juice (optional)
lettuce or *other green salad leaves to garnish (optional)*

❋ Cut the tomato (or tomatoes) in half, scoop out the soft centre and seeds (you could add this to a pasta sauce or soup). Turn the tomatoes upside-down to drain.

❋ Mix together the cottage cheese, fromage frais, and herbs. Season to taste with salt and freshly milled black pepper and lemon juice if you like.

❋ Stuff each tomato half with the cheese mixture. Serve alone or on a bed of lettuce or other leaves.

COTTAGE CHEESE AND FRUIT SALAD

All these ingredients are so low in calories that you can go to town and really eat your fill.

SERVES 1

*a selection of fruit, e.g. apples, pears, grapes, kiwi, mango, papaya
(pawpaw), melon, peaches
a little lime or lemon juice
lettuce leaves or other green salad leaves
2–3 oz (50–75 g) cottage cheese*

✻ Prepare and slice the fruit and sprinkle with the lime or lemon juice.
✻ Make a base of the lettuce leaves and put the cottage cheese in the middle. Arrange the sliced fruit attractively around the cottage cheese and serve.

SMOKED MACKEREL PÂTÉ

SERVES 2

*2 oz (50 g) smoked mackerel fillet
4 oz (100 g) low-fat soft cheese
1 tablespoon lemon juice
1 tablespoon chopped onion
freshly milled black pepper*

✻ Skin the mackerel and flake it. Add the cheese, lemon juice, onion and pepper to taste. Blend all ingredients together until they form a smooth paste.
✻ Chill thoroughly and serve with wholemeal toast or 'free' salad (see p. 218).

QUICK GRAVAD LAX

This pickled salmon is a Scandinavian speciality and a cheap alternative to smoked salmon. This is a quick way of making a small quantity of it. The traditional recipes often call for 'half a salmon' and take a couple of days to make. (The salt and sugar, by the way, are mostly discarded at the end.) You need salmon fillet – cut horizontally – not salmon steak for this recipe.

This recipe also comes with a low-calorie version of the traditional sauce.

SERVES 2

1 × 4–5 oz (100–150 g) boneless salmon fillet
1 tablespoon finely chopped fresh dill
2 teaspoons salt
2 teaspoons sugar
2 teaspoons vodka or brandy (optional)
fresh dill to garnish (optional)

✳ Skin the fish by first lifting a corner with a sharp knife. Once you have got a grip, carefully peel the skin off. If you haven't done it before, this is easier than you think. Feel along for any small bones and remove them with a pair of tweezers if necessary.

✳ Mix together the dill, salt, sugar and the vodka or brandy (if you are using any). Spread this mixture all over the salmon. Place it in a small dish in which it just fits and cover with cling film.

✳ Refrigerate for 6–12 hours, turning now and again. Liquid is produced and if your dish is small enough, it will cover the salmon. If not, turn more frequently.

✳ Wipe or wash off the marinade and slice the salmon into small, very thin, strips. Serve with salad (any salad ingredients on the 'free' list on p. 188) and the following sauce. Garnish with more fresh dill if you like.

DILL AND MUSTARD SAUCE FOR GRAVAD LAX

SERVES 2

1 tablespoon finely chopped fresh dill
1/4–1/2 teaspoon Dijon mustard
1/2 teaspoon caster sugar
1 tablespoon 8% fromage frais (see p. 90)

❋ Whisk all the ingredients together and serve at the side of the salmon.

SPANISH OMELETTE

SERVES 1

1 tablespoon chopped onion
1/4–1/2 red or green pepper, de-seeded and chopped
2 oz (50 g) mushrooms, chopped
4 oz (100 g) tomatoes, chopped
2 oz (50 g) cold cooked potato, diced
2 oz (50 g) cooked peas
2 eggs (see p. 89)

❋ In a heavy, non-stick frying-pan, 'dry fry' (see p. 86) the onion and green or red pepper until soft.
❋ Add the mushroom, tomatoes, potatoes and peas and heat.
❋ Beat the eggs and add to the mixture. Cook until set.

MUSHROOM OMELETTE

SERVES 1

2–4 oz (50–100 g) mushrooms, sliced
2 eggs (see p. 89)
1 tablespoon skimmed milk from allowance
salt and freshly milled black pepper

* 'Dry-fry' the mushrooms until soft. Set aside until cool.
* Lightly whisk together the eggs, milk and seasoning to taste. Add the cooked mushrooms.
* Heat a heavy, non-stick frying-pan – about 7–8 inches (18–20 cm) across – on a medium heat. When it's hot, add the eggs and stir two or three times with a wooden spoon, bringing the setting egg from the edge to the centre and allowing the liquid egg to flow onto the pan's surface.
* Leave the omelette on a medium heat for a minute or so until it is set but still slightly moist.
* Fold the omelette and turn out onto a hot plate.

COTTAGE CHEESE AND CHIVE OMELETTE

SERVES 1

2 tablespoons cottage cheese
1 tablespoon 8% fromage frais or Greek yoghurt (see p. 90)
1 tablespoon finely chopped fresh chives
salt and freshly milled black pepper
2 eggs (see p. 89)
1 tablespoon skimmed milk

* Thoroughly mix together the cottage cheese, fromage frais or yoghurt and the chives. Season this mixture.
* Lightly whisk together the eggs and milk. Season.
* Heat a heavy non-stick frying-pan – about 7–8 inches (18–20 cm) across – on a medium heat. When it's hot, add the eggs and stir two or three times with a wooden spoon, bringing the setting egg from the edge to the centre and allowing the liquid egg to flow onto the pan's surface.
* Distribute the cottage cheese filling along the middle of the omelette and leave the omelette on a medium heat for a minute or so until the filling is warm and the omelette is set but still slightly moist.
* Fold the omelette and turn out onto a hot plate.

251

FRITTATA

This solid Italian omelette is good hot or cold.

SERVES 1

½ small onion, finely chopped
1 clove garlic, peeled and finely chopped (optional)
2 eggs (see p. 89)
1 tablespoon skimmed milk
1 tablespoon finely chopped fresh basil
salt and freshly milled black pepper
2 ripe tomatoes, quartered (skinned if preferred)

* In a heavy non-stick frying-pan, about 6–7 inches (15–18 cm) in diameter, 'dry-fry' (see p. 86) the onion and garlic until they are soft.
* Whisk together the eggs and milk. Stir in the basil and season.
* Arrange the quartered tomatoes over the onion and garlic and pour the egg mixture over them.
  Cook on a gentle heat until the omelette is well set.
* Turn over and continue to cook for a minute or two.
* Alternatively, place the frying-pan under a pre-heated grill for 1–2 minutes to set the top. This may be easier!

FRESH MIXED HERB OMELETTE

You can use any combination of fresh herbs for this omelette but perhaps the best is a mixture of parsley, chives, chervil and tarragon.

SERVES 1

2 eggs (see p. 89)
1 tablespoon 8% fromage frais or Greek yoghurt (see p. 90)
2 tablespoons finely chopped fresh mixed herbs
salt and freshly milled black pepper

* Lightly whisk together the eggs and fromage frais or Greek yoghurt. Stir in the herbs and season.
* Heat a heavy non-stick frying-pan – about 7–8 inches (18–20 cm) across – on a medium heat. When it's hot, add the eggs and stir two or three times with a wooden spoon, bringing the setting egg from the edge to the centre and allowing the liquid egg to flow onto the pan's surface.
* Leave the omelette on a medium heat for a minute or so until it is set but still slightly moist.
* Fold the omelette and turn out onto a hot plate.

PASTA AND RICE

SPAGHETTI WITH MUSHROOM SAUCE

If you prefer, you can always double the quantities for the sauce in this recipe and freeze one portion as a handy stand-by.

SERVES 1

1 clove garlic, peeled and finely chopped
4 oz (100 g) large open mushrooms, diced
1 x 7-oz (200-g) tin tomatoes or 3 medium tomatoes, diced
(skinned if preferred)
½ tablespoon chopped fresh oregano or ½ teaspoon dried oregano
½ tablespoon chopped fresh parsley
salt and freshly milled black pepper
4 oz (100 g) dried spaghetti or other pasta

* 'Dry-fry' (see p. 86) the garlic in a heavy non-stick frying-pan for 1–2 minutes. Add the diced mushrooms and fry for a further 1–2 minutes. Then add the tomatoes and the herbs. Simmer for 15–20 minutes. Season to taste.
* Meanwhile cook the spaghetti in a pan of lightly salted boiling water for 7–8 minutes until cooked but still firm. Drain.
* Toss the cooked, drained spaghetti with the mushroom sauce and serve, sprinkled with a little more chopped parsley if wished.

SPAGHETTI WITH BROCCOLI

Well-cooked broccoli has a melting quality which makes a tasty pasta sauce.

SERVES 1

1 clove garlic, peeled and finely chopped
6 oz (175 g) broccoli, fresh or frozen and thawed
3 oz (75 g) dried spaghetti or other pasta
salt and freshly milled black pepper
2 teaspoons freshly grated Parmesan cheese

✳ 'Dry-fry' (see p. 86) the garlic for 1–2 minutes in a heavy non-stick frying-pan. Finely dice the broccoli and add that to the garlic. Stir for another 1–2 minutes. Add 4–5 tablespoons of water and stir vigorously if the broccoli begins to stick. Simmer gently for 10–15 minutes until the broccoli is soft and breaking up, adding another couple of tablespoons of water when the pan is dry. The idea is to be left with soft broccoli with very little liquid.

✳ Cook the spaghetti in a pan of lightly salted boiling water for 7–8 minutes or until it's cooked but still firm.

✳ Drain the spaghetti and toss with the broccoli. Season with salt and freshly milled black pepper. Serve on a heated plate and sprinkle with the Parmesan cheese.

SPAGHETTI WITH FRESH TOMATO AND BASIL SAUCE

This is a pleasing combination of hot pasta and cold sauce and is so simple and quick to make. Instead of using spaghetti you could serve the sauce on tagliatelle or a similar pasta.

SERVES 1

3 oz (75 g) dried spaghetti
2 large or 3 medium tomatoes
1 teaspoon wine vinegar or squeeze of lemon juice
1 heaped teaspoon finely chopped fresh basil
salt and freshly milled black pepper

* Cook the spaghetti in a pan of lightly salted boiling water for 8–9 minutes or until it's cooked but still firm.
* Meanwhile, finely chop the tomatoes into the smallest possible dice – ¼ inch (5 mm) or so.
* Mix the chopped tomato, wine vinegar and basil in a bowl and season to taste.
* Toss the cold tomato and basil mixture with the hot drained pasta and serve immediately.

TAGLIATELLE AL LIMONE (NOODLES WITH LEMON SAUCE)

SERVES 1

2–3 oz (50–75 g) tagliatelle or spaghetti
zest and juice of ½ lemon
½–1 clove garlic, peeled and finely chopped (optional)
2 tablespoons Greek yoghurt
¼ oz (10 g) freshly grated Parmesan cheese
salt and freshly milled black pepper

❋ Cook the pasta in lightly salted boiling water until cooked but still firm.

❋ Add the lemon juice, zest and garlic (if using) to the yoghurt and heat gently. (Unlike normal low-fat yoghurt, Greek-style yoghurt does not separate when heated gently but *do not boil*.)

❋ When the pasta is cooked, drain well and add to the lemon sauce. Mix well. Serve on a heated plate and sprinkle with the Parmesan and pepper to taste.

MACARONI COTTAGE CHEESE

SERVES 2

½ oz (15 g) sunflower margarine
½ oz (15 g) flour
5 fl oz (150 ml) skimmed milk
4 oz (100 g) cottage cheese
handful of chopped fresh chives
1 teaspoon English mustard or 2 teaspoons French mustard
1 oz (25 g) strong Cheddar or Parmesan cheese, grated
4 oz (100 g) macaroni
salt and freshly milled black pepper

❋ Melt the margarine in a pan. Add the flour and stir over a gentle heat for 2 minutes.

❋ Take the pan off the heat and gradually stir in the milk. Replace the pan on the heat and stir until the sauce has thickened.

❋ Add the cottage cheese, chives, mustard and half the cheese. Season to taste.

❋ Boil the macaroni for 8–10 minutes until cooked but still firm. Drain and place in an ovenproof dish.

❋ Pour the sauce over the macaroni, top with the remaining cheese, and place under the grill until golden.

PASTA SHAPES IN TOMATO SAUCE

This amount of sauce makes two generous portions with 6 oz (175 g) pasta as a main course. The same amount with 6 oz (175 g) pasta will serve three people who want to lose weight more quickly! Freeze individual portions of this sauce to rustle up quick meals when you're busy. To vary the sauce you can also add 1 finely chopped red or green pepper when cooking the onion and garlic.

SERVES 2

1 onion, finely chopped

1–2 cloves garlic, peeled and finely chopped

1 × 14-oz (400-g) tin chopped tomatoes

½ teaspoon dried oregano or 1 tablespoon finely chopped fresh
oregano or fresh basil

salt and freshly milled black pepper

4–6 oz (100–175 g) dried pasta shapes such as shells, bows or
quills

½ oz (15 g) freshly grated Parmesan cheese

❋ 'Dry fry' (see p. 86) the onion and garlic in a heavy non-stick saucepan. When soft add the tomatoes and dried herbs, if using them. Simmer for 10 minutes. Add fresh herbs now, if using them and season to taste.

❋ Cook pasta for 12–15 minutes as directed on the packet. Drain well and add the sauce.

❋ Stir, serve on heated plates and sprinkle with Parmesan.

PASTA WITH CREAMY MUSHROOMS
....

You can use any type of pasta for this dish from tagliatelle to pasta shells or quills.

SERVES 1

2–3 oz (50–75 g) dried pasta
1 clove garlic, peeled and finely chopped (optional)
3 oz (75 g) mushrooms
1 tablespoon Greek yoghurt or 8% fromage frais (see p. 90)
2 teaspoons finely chopped fresh parsley
¼ oz (10 g) freshly grated Parmesan cheese

❋ Cook the pasta in lightly salted water until it is cooked but still firm.

❋ 'Dry fry' (see p. 86) the garlic (if using) and mushrooms in a heavy non-stick pan until the mushrooms are very soft. Add the pasta to the mushrooms with the yoghurt or fromage frais and mix well. Stir in the parsley.

❋ Serve on a heated plate and sprinkle with the Parmesan.

BROCCOLI RISOTTO

This is an inviting cream and green colour and the well-cooked broccoli makes a melting sauce. You could use vegetable stock instead of water if you prefer.

SERVES 1

6 oz (175 g) broccoli, fresh or frozen
½ small onion, finely chopped
1 clove garlic, peeled and finely chopped (optional)
3 oz (75 g) white round rice (preferably Arborio or Italian risotto)
1 tablespoon freshly grated Parmesan cheese
salt and freshly milled black pepper

* Trim the broccoli and dice the stalk and florets into ½-inch (1-cm) pieces.
* 'Dry fry' (see p. 86) the onion and garlic in a heavy non-stick frying-pan until soft but not at all coloured.
* Meanwhile, boil up a kettle of water or have a pan with a pint or so of water or stock simmering.
* Add the rice to the onion and garlic and stir for about a minute, then add the broccoli and stir for a further minute.
* Start adding the hot water a ladle or a cupful at a time. Stir well and keep the rice bubbling gently. As the rice becomes dryish, add more water.
* Keep stirring frequently and adding a ladle of water until the rice is cooked but still a little firm in the centre. This should take 25–35 minutes. There should still be a spoonful or so of liquid as a sauce.
* Add half of the Parmesan cheese, stir and season to taste.
* Serve on a heated plate sprinkled with the rest of the cheese.

MUSHROOM RISOTTO

For this delicious risotto it's much better if you can find the dried cèpes or Porcini mushrooms: they're expensive, but a little goes a long way.

SERVES 1

½ small onion, finely chopped
1 clove garlic, peeled and finely chopped
3 oz (75 g) white round rice (preferably Arborio or Italian risotto)
6 oz (175 g) large open flat mushrooms, finely diced or 4 oz
(100 g) large open flat mushrooms and ¼ oz (10 g) dried cèpes (or
Porcini mushrooms)
½ glass dry white wine (optional)
1 tablespoon finely grated Parmesan cheese
salt and freshly milled black pepper
finely chopped fresh parsley to garnish (optional)

❋ If you are using dried cèpes or Porcini mushrooms, soak them for 15–20 minutes in a little boiling water, drain them reserving the liquid, and finely chop.

❋ 'Dry fry' (see p. 86) the onion and garlic in a large, heavy non-stick frying-pan until very soft but not at all coloured.

❋ Have ready about a pint (600 ml) of water simmering in another pan. (You could use vegetable stock if you prefer.)

❋ Add the rice and 'dry fry' with the onion and garlic for about a minute, stirring all the time. Add the mushrooms (including the cèpes or Porcini mushrooms, if using) and stir for another minute. Add the strained liquid from the dried mushrooms if you are using them.

❋ Add the wine, if using, and stir well.

❋ Now add the simmering water to the contents of the pan, about a ladleful at a time. Stir the rice frequently and ensure the water is always gently bubbling. The idea is to keep adding the water as the rice becomes dry. It's worth the extra trouble, as the result is different – and much better – than adding all the water at once.

❋ When the rice is cooked, but still a little firm in the centre (after about 25–35 minutes), add half the Parmesan cheese, stir and season to taste.

❋ Serve on a heated plate garnished with parsley if wished. Sprinkle with the remaining cheese.

VEGETARIAN DISHES

POTATO AND MUSHROOM GRATIN

Gratin dauphinois *is a wickedly fattening French gratin of potatoes; this is based on the same idea and is rich and filling – and still slimming! Check the instructions on your diet plan for the quantity of potatoes you should use.*

SERVES 1

7–9 oz (200–250 g) potatoes, preferably yellow, waxy ones
2 tablespoons 8% fromage frais (see p. 90)
2 tablespoons skimmed milk
1 clove garlic, peeled
4 oz (100 g) large flat mushrooms, wiped and thinly sliced
1 teaspoon freshly grated Parmesan cheese (optional)
salt and freshly milled black pepper

* Pre-heat the oven to gas mark 4, 350°F (180°C).
* Peel the potatoes and slice them into thin even rounds (about the thickness of a two-pence coin).
* Put the fromage frais in a bowl and whisk it lightly with the skimmed milk. Crush the garlic clove to a paste with a little salt and stir into the mixture. Then add the potato slices and turn over and over until they are all coated.
* In an earthenware ovenproof dish, place layers of overlapping slices of potatoes, alternating with the mushrooms and ending with a layer of potatoes. Sprinkle on the Parmesan if using and season to taste.
* Bake the gratin in the oven for 50 minutes or until the potatoes are soft and the top is browned. (Cover with a piece of foil if it starts to brown too quickly.)

BARBECUED TOFU WITH RICE

···

Tofu – made from soya beans – has no taste itself but does have a great ability to pick up other flavours. For this delicious dish, you need the firm tofu which comes in a block, not the soft, or silken, tofu.

SERVES 1
1 tablespoon tomato ketchup or tomato purée
1 tablespoon wine or cider vinegar
1 tablespoon soy sauce
1 tablespoon dry sherry or dry vermouth or water
2 tablespoons orange juice
2 cloves garlic
1-inch (2.5-cm) piece fresh root ginger
4 oz (100 g) firm tofu
2½ oz (65 g) brown rice

❋ Whisk together the tomato ketchup or purée, vinegar, soy sauce, sherry, vermouth or water and orange juice.

❋ Peel and slice the garlic and root ginger and add them to this sauce mixture.

❋ Cut the tofu into slices of about 3 × ¾ × ¾ inches (7.5 × 2 × 2 cm). Place them in the sauce mixture and mix well.

❋ Let the tofu slices marinate in the mixture for at least 6 and up to 24 hours.

❋ When you're ready to eat, simmer the brown rice, in salted water, for 35–40 minutes until tender.

❋ Drain the tofu slices, and keep the marinade mixture. Grill the tofu on a sheet of foil under the highest heat for 8–10 minutes. Turn them 2 or 3 times during this time. They are ready when the edges just begin to char.

❋ Meanwhile, heat the marinade mixture in a small pan.

❋ Serve the tofu with the drained rice and marinade sauce.

CAULIFLOWER CHEESE

This is a tasty low-calorie version of an old favourite. Because it's part of your main meal, I've suggested in this instance using full-fat Cheddar.

SERVES 1
½ cauliflower
5 lf oz (150 ml) White sauce (see p. 345)
½–1 teaspoon Dijon mustard (optional)
1 oz (25 g) Cheddar, finely grated (vegetarian, if you prefer)
salt and freshly milled black pepper

❋ Steam or simmer or microwave the cauliflower until it is tender but still firm.
❋ Make up the White sauce, whisk in the mustard (if using) and three-quarters of the grated cheese. Season to taste.
❋ Drain the cauliflower well and arrange, in two or three pieces if necessary, in a warmed heatproof dish. Pour over the sauce and scatter the remaining cheese on top.
❋ Brown under a pre-heated grill.

CHICK PEA CURRY

This makes a satisfying curry and is quick if you use tinned chick peas. Serve with a portion of Minty cucumber salad (see p. 323). Instead of the individual dried spices you could use 2 teaspoons of curry powder.

SERVES 1
3½ oz (90 g) dried chick peas, soaked overnight or 1 × 14-oz
(400-g) tin chick peas
1 small onion, finely chopped
1–2 cloves of garlic, peeled and finely chopped
1-inch (2.5-cm) piece fresh root ginger, peeled and finely chopped

1 fresh green chilli, de-seeded and finely chopped (optional)
2 teaspoons ground coriander
1 teaspoon ground cumin
½ teaspoon turmeric
2 large or 3 medium tomatoes, finely chopped (skinned if
preferred) or 1 × 7-oz (200-g) tin tomatoes
squeeze of lemon juice
salt
1 tablespoon low-fat yoghurt (optional)

＊ If you're using dried chick peas, cook the soaked chick peas in fresh water for an hour or so until they are tender. Drain, but reserve the cooking water. In the same way, drain the tinned chick peas (if using) and keep the liquid.

＊ 'Dry fry' (see p. 86) the onion, garlic, ginger and chilli (if using) in a heavy non-stick frying-pan for 3–4 minutes until they are soft and browning. Stir in the spices and stir and fry for a minute or two more. Add the chopped tomatoes, lemon juice, and a little of the liquid from the tin of chick peas or the cooking water. Stir well, scraping the bottom of the pan with a wooden spoon.

＊ Now add the chick peas. Stir and simmer for 10–15 minutes until the curry is nice and thick. Add a little more chick pea liquid or cooking water if it seems dry.

＊ Season with salt to taste, and, off the heat, stir in the yoghurt if using. Serve immediately.

NOTE If you cook 5 oz (150 g) brown rice separately and serve this with the curry, there will be enough for 2 servings.

CHICK PEA PAPRIKA

SERVES 2
4 oz (100 g) brown rice
1 onion, finely chopped
1 clove garlic, peeled and finely chopped
1 small red pepper, de-seeded and cut into strips
2 teaspoons paprika
1 × 14-oz (400-g) tin chick peas, drained
1 × 14-oz (400-g) tin chopped tomatoes
2 tablespoons natural low-fat yoghurt (see p. 90)
salt and freshly milled black pepper

* Cook the brown rice in water; it will take approximately 40 minutes.
* 'Dry fry' (see p. 86) the onion and garlic in a heavy non-stick saucepan until soft. Add the red pepper strips and cook for a further few minutes. Add the paprika and stir well.
* Add the drained chick peas and the chopped tomatoes. Simmer for 15–20 minutes or until the rice is ready. Season to taste.
* Put the yoghurt on top of the chick pea paprika just before serving (having removed the saucepan from the heat). Drain the rice and serve with the chick peas.

VEGETABLE STIR-FRY

This is very quick and easy to make and you can vary it endlessly (see below).

SERVES 1
1 small onion
1 red, yellow or green pepper, de-seeded
2 courgettes

1-inch (2.5-cm) piece fresh root ginger, peeled and finely chopped
or grated
1–2 cloves garlic, peeled and finely chopped
2 oz (50 g) closed cap mushrooms, wiped and thickly sliced
1 tablespoon soy sauce
1 tablespoon orange juice or 1 tablespoon tomato ketchup or
tomato purée
1 tablespoon dry white wine or dry white vermouth
1–2 teaspoons wine or cider vinegar

❋ Chop the onion, pepper and courgettes into bite-size pieces.
❋ 'Dry fry' (see p. 86) the ginger, garlic and onion in a large non-stick frying-pan for 2–3 minutes until they begin to soften. Add the peppers and courgettes and stir-fry for a further 2 minutes. Add the mushrooms and continue to stir-fry for another 1–2 minutes until the vegetables are as you like them (preferably still crunchy!).
❋ Meanwhile mix together the other ingredients according to which alternatives you have chosen. When the vegetables are ready, stir in this sauce, mix well, and let it bubble for 30–40 seconds. Serve.

NOTE

✱ Remember the technique (p.86) of adding a tablespoon of water at a time and stirring vigorously if the vegetables start to stick.
✱ On the whole, a frying-pan is better than a wok (see p. 87).
✱ You can vary this stir-fry dish by adding or substituting any of the following vegetables (sliced or in bite-size pieces): carrots, leeks, swedes, turnips, broccoli, cauliflower, cabbage, Chinese cabbage, French or runner beans (see p. 218 for suggested quantities).

MUSHROOM, OLIVE AND CAPER PIZZA
·······································

Don't be put off by the fact that this calls for yeast. Using easy-blend yeast is simple. (Always mix it with the flour before adding any liquid.) I find the dough is ready by the time I've prepared the other ingredients, so the whole thing is quite quick.

SERVES 1
a good pinch of salt
1 scant flat teaspoon easy-blend yeast
3 oz (75 g) strong plain flour
warm water to mix
3 medium tomatoes or 7-oz (200-g) tin chopped tomatoes, drained
1 tablespoon fresh oregano or ½ teaspoon dried oregano
1 clove garlic, peeled and finely chopped (optional)
salt and freshly milled black pepper
2 oz (50 g) mushrooms, thinly sliced
½–1 tablespoon capers
6 black olives, stoned

* Pre-heat the oven to gas mark 6, 400°F (200°C).
* Mix the salt and yeast with the flour and add just enough hand-hot water to blend into a workable dough (this takes 10–15 seconds in a food processor). Knead the dough between the floured palms of your hands for 2 or 3 minutes or process for another minute or so. Put the dough in a floured polythene bag and leave in a warm place while you prepare the vegetables. Try to leave it for 15–20 minutes.
* If you are using fresh tomatoes, peel and chop them and leave them to drain in a sieve. Mix the oregano and garlic, plus salt and freshly milled black pepper, into the chopped tomatoes or the drained tinned tomatoes.
* Roll or press out the dough to about a 10-inch (25-cm) round. Place it on a very lightly oiled baking sheet or foil.
* Arrange the sliced mushrooms over the pizza and then evenly distribute the tomato mixture on top. Sprinkle over the capers and arrange the olives on the pizza.

❊ Bake for about 25 minutes until the dough is cooked and the edges are crisp and browning.

VEGETABLE CHILLI

If you want to eat just one helping, the other half will freeze well.

SERVES 2
1 small onion, chopped
1–2 cloves garlic, peeled and chopped
1–2 fresh green chillies or ¼–½ teaspoon cayenne
2 sticks of celery, de-stringed and chopped
2 carrots, chopped
1 small red and 1 small green pepper, de-seeded and chopped
1–2 teaspoons paprika
1 teaspoon ground cumin
½ teaspoon dried oregano
3 medium tomatoes, peeled and chopped or 1 × 7-oz (200-g) tin
chopped tomatoes
5 oz (150 g) dried red kidney beans, soaked overnight or 1 × 14-oz
(400-g) tin red kidney beans, drained
salt and freshly milled black pepper

❊ If you're using dried beans, discard the soaking water and bring them to the boil in a pan of fresh water. Boil fast for 10 minutes, then simmer until soft. Drain and set aside.

❊ Stir-fry the onion, garlic and fresh chilli (if using) until they are soft. Add the celery, carrots, and peppers and stir and fry for another couple of minutes. Then stir in the cayenne, if you are using it, the paprika, cumin and oregano.

❊ Mix in the tomatoes (and a little water if you are using fresh tomatoes) and stir well, ensuring that anything sticking is stirred in. Lastly, add the kidney beans.

❊ Simmer for 10–15 minutes. Season to taste.

PEPPERS STUFFED WITH BULGAR PILAF

You can of course vary the mixture of herbs used in this dish.

SERVES 1

½ medium onion, finely chopped

1–2 cloves garlic, peeled and finely chopped

2 oz (50 g) bulgar wheat (burghul, pourgouri or cracked wheat)

2 teaspoons raisins or sultanas

1–2 tablespoons finely chopped fresh parsley, chives and dill

½ teaspoon ground cinnamon (optional)

salt and freshly milled black pepper

1 large red, yellow or green pepper

1 tablespoon tomato purée

1–2 teaspoons wine or cider vinegar or lemon juice

1–2 tablespoons low-fat natural yoghurt (optional)

❋ Pre-heat the oven to gas mark 4, 350°F (180°C).

❋ 'Dry fry' (see p. 86) the onion and garlic until soft but not coloured. Add the bulgar and raisins or sultanas and mix well. Add 5 fl oz (150 ml) of hot water, stir and simmer for 3–4 minutes until the water is almost absorbed and the bulgar is swollen and tender. Add more water as needed to swell the bulgar. Don't end up with a mixture which is completely dry. Stir in the fresh herbs, and cinnamon, if using, season and set to one side.

❋ Cut the pepper in half, remove the core, seeds and white pith. Place in a small ovenproof dish, open side up. Stuff the pepper halves with the bulgar pilaf.

❋ Mix the tomato purée with the vinegar or lemon juice and 4 tablespoons of water. Pour over and around the peppers.

❋ Bake the peppers in the oven for 25–30 minutes or until they are cooked. Serve with the natural yoghurt if you like.

NOTE You could use 2 or 3 courgettes instead of a pepper. Halve them, scrape out the middle of the flesh and stuff them.

VEGETARIAN MOUSSAKA

If you liked, you could divide this in two separate portions and freeze one of them.

SERVES 2

2 aubergines
1 onion, finely chopped
2 cloves garlic, peeled and finely chopped
1–2 sticks celery, de-stringed and finely chopped (optional)
1–2 carrots, finely chopped (optional)
6 oz (175 g) large flat open mushrooms, chopped
1 × 14-oz (400-g) tin chopped tomatoes
1 tablespoon tomato purée
1 tablespoon fresh oregano or 1 teaspoon dried oregano
salt and freshly milled black pepper
1 egg
4 tablespoons Greek yoghurt
2 tablespoons skimmed milk
1 oz (25 g) Cheddar, finely grated (vegetarian if wished)

* Pre-heat the oven to gas mark 4, 350°F (180°C).
* Take the stalks off the aubergines and cut them into ¼-inch (½-cm) slices. Lay them out and sprinkle with salt. Leave them to stand while you prepare the other ingredients. Turn them now and again. Then wash and pat dry. (This draws out any bitter juices from the aubergines; I find nowadays that most aubergines are not bitter even without this process, but some still are, so on the whole, it's worth doing. It also ensures that the finished dish is not watery.)
* Meanwhile, 'dry fry' (see p. 86) the onion and garlic until soft, then, if using, add the celery and carrots and continue to stir and fry for another couple of minutes. Then add the mushrooms and fry them until their juices begin to run.
* Add the tomatoes, tomato purée, and oregano and stir well. Simmer for 10–15 minutes until some of the moisture has

been drained off and the mixture has thickened a little. Season to taste.

* With a piece of oiled kitchen paper, lightly grease a suitable ovenproof dish. Place alternate layers of aubergine slices and tomato mixture in the dish, ending with aubergine.

* Whisk together the egg, Greek yoghurt, skimmed milk and half of the cheese. Season. Pour this mixture over the aubergines. Sprinkle over the rest of the cheese.

* Bake in the oven for about 30 minutes or until the aubergines are soft and the top is browned.

FISH

STUFFED BAKED TROUT

SERVES 2

2 × 6–7 oz (175–200 g) trout, fresh or frozen and thawed
1½ oz (40 g) fresh wholemeal breadcrumbs
2 oz (50 g) mushrooms, finely diced
1 tablespoon finely chopped fresh parsley
1 clove garlic, peeled and finely chopped (optional)
grated zest and juice of 1 lemon
salt and freshly milled black pepper
½ teaspoon polyunsaturated oil (e.g. sunflower)

* Pre-heat the oven to gas mark 4, 350°F (180°C).
* Clean the trout and dry with kitchen paper.
* In a bowl, mix together the breadcrumbs, mushrooms, parsley, garlic, the zest and half of the lemon juice. Season.
* Stuff this mixture into the body of the trout.
* Lightly oil a large sheet of kitchen foil, large enough to hold both trout comfortably. Place the trout side by side, head to tail on the foil, pour over the remaining lemon juice, fold the foil into a parcel shape and tightly seal the joints by folding over several times.
* Bake the trout in the oven for 25–30 minutes. Uncover after 25 minutes and check if it is ready by inserting a knife gently near the backbone. The flesh should come away easily.
* Serve the trout on heated plates, pouring the juices over.

COLD TROUT MARINATED IN ORANGE

This is based on an Italian method of using left-over fried fish. It certainly doesn't taste like left-overs!

SERVES 1

1 × 6–7 oz (175–200 g) trout, fresh or frozen and thawed
3 tablespoons orange juice or juice and grated zest of 1 orange
juice of ½ lemon
2 tablespoons white wine or white vermouth or water
couple sprigs of parsley
sprig of fresh thyme or a small pinch dried thyme
1 clove of garlic, peeled and halved
salt and freshly milled black pepper
parsley and a slice or two of fresh orange to garnish

❋ Clean the trout and dry with kitchen paper. Then 'dry fry' (see p. 86) it in a heavy non-stick frying-pan over a medium heat for 7–8 minutes until it is just cooked. Don't overcook. Alternatively, grill the trout under a moderate heat for the same length of time. Set aside to cool.

❋ Meanwhile, prepare the marinade. In a small pan boil together the orange juice (and zest if using) and lemon juice, the wine or water, the herbs and the garlic. Simmer for a couple of minutes or until it is reduced by half. Season.

❋ When the trout is cool enough to handle, remove the skin with a small knife. Place the trout in a small deep dish and pour over the warm marinade.

❋ Serve the trout when it is cold, garnished with the parsley and orange slices if using. The flavour is better if it hasn't been refrigerated, but if you do refrigerate (overnight, say) bring to room temperature before serving.

TROUT WITH CUCUMBER SAUCE

SERVES 1

1 × 6–7 oz (175–200 g) trout, fresh or frozen and thawed
1 tablespoon 8% fromage frais (see p. 90) and 1 tablespoon low-
fat natural yoghurt or 1 tablespoon 1% fromage frais and 1
tablespoon Greek yoghurt
2-inch (5-cm) piece cucumber, finely diced
salt and freshly milled black pepper
squeeze of lemon juice

* Clean the trout and dry with kitchen paper. Then 'dry fry'
(see p. 86) or grill it for 7–8 minutes until the skin is
browning and the flesh cooked, but still moist.
* Meanwhile, whisk together the fromage frais and yoghurt,
stir in the cucumber. Season with salt, pepper and lemon juice.
* Serve the hot trout with the cold sauce.

GRILLED TROUT WITH BACON

*This is based on a traditional Welsh dish – brithyll â chig moch –
and you'll find the bacon gives the trout a lovely flavour.*

SERVES 1

1 oz (25 g) or 1 thin rasher of back bacon, smoked or unsmoked
1 × 6–7 oz (175–200 g) trout, fresh or frozen and thawed
lemon quarter and sprig of parsley to garnish

* Trim all the fat from the bacon and cut it into 3 long strips.
Clean the trout and dry it with kitchen paper. Then wind
the strips of bacon around the trout.
Grill the trout under a hot pre-heated grill for 7–8 minutes,
turning once, until the flesh is cooked and the bacon and the
skin are browning.
* Serve garnished with the lemon and parsley.

GRILLED COD WITH PARSLEY SAUCE

If you prefer, you can always make this simple dish with an equivalent quantity of haddock instead of cod.

SERVES 1

*5 oz (150 g) cod steak or fillet, fresh or frozen
1 quantity of Parsley sauce (see p. 345)
sprig of parsley to garnish*

❋ Grill the fish on a lightly oiled piece of foil (see p. 87) for 6–8 minutes if cooking from fresh or about 20 minutes from frozen, turning once.
❋ Serve with the sauce and garnish with parsley.

GRILLED HADDOCK WITH FROMAGE FRAIS

The fromage frais gives a very appetising brown colour to the fish and keeps it moist. It does get brown quite quickly so watch it carefully. Instead of haddock you could use any other white fish if you prefer.

SERVES 1

*5 oz (150 g) haddock fillet or steak, fresh or frozen
1 tablespoon 8% fromage frais (see p. 90)
sprig of parsley and a lemon quarter to garnish*

❋ Grill the haddock on a lightly oiled piece of foil (see p. 87) for 3–4 minutes if cooking from fresh or 8–10 minutes from frozen. Turn over and spread the fromage frais over the fish. Grill for a similar time again until the fish is cooked and the fromage frais is browned.
❋ Serve garnished with the parsley and lemon.

HADDOCK WITH YELLOW PEPPER SAUCE

You could use any white fish for this recipe. Either all or just one or two of the herbs may be used if you prefer.

SERVES 1

10 fl oz (300 ml) water or half water and half wine (or dry
vermouth)
sprig of fennel
sprig of thyme
sprig of parsley
small bay leaf
a few peppercorns
5 oz (150 g) haddock fillet
1 clove garlic, peeled and finely chopped
1 large yellow pepper, de-seeded and chopped
1 tablespoon Greek yoghurt
salt and freshly milled black pepper
squeeze of lemon juice
fresh fennel to garnish (optional)

❊ Boil the water, or water and wine, with the herbs and peppercorns for 5 minutes. Strain and poach the fish in the flavoured water for 5 minutes or so until it is just cooked. Drain and keep warm, reserving the liquid. Then boil this rapidly until it has reduced by about two-thirds.

❊ Meanwhile, 'dry fry' (see p. 86) the garlic and pepper for about 5 minutes or until soft.

❊ Put the pepper and garlic and the reduced stock into a liquidiser or food processor and process until smooth. Turn out into a clean pan and re-heat gently. Off the heat, whisk in the Greek yoghurt, season with salt, pepper and a squeeze of lemon juice.

❊ Pour the sauce over a heated plate. Place the fish neatly in the middle and garnish with some fresh fennel if you like.

FISHERMAN'S PIE

If you are in a hurry, you could also make this with instant mashed potato.

SERVES 1

5–7 oz (150–200 g) potatoes
1 tablespoon 8% fromage frais (see p. 90)
1 tablespoon skimmed milk
salt and freshly milled black pepper
5 oz (150 g) cod or haddock fillet
5 fl oz (150 ml) skimmed milk
½ oz (15 g) plain flour
½ oz (15 g) low-fat spread
squeeze of lemon juice
1 tablespoon finely chopped fresh parsley (optional)
1 oz (25 g) prawns or 1 teaspoon anchovy essence (optional)

* Pre-heat the oven to gas mark 4, 350°F (180°C).
* Peel the potatoes and simmer in water until they are cooked. Drain, mash and stir in the fromage frais and tablespoon of skimmed milk. Season to taste.
* Meanwhile, poach the cod or haddock in the 5 fl oz (150 ml) milk until cooked. Drain, keeping the milk. Flake the fish.
* When the milk is cold, make a white sauce with it using the flour and low-fat spread (see p. 345 for method).
* Season the sauce with salt, freshly milled black pepper, lemon juice and add the parsley if using. Also stir in the prawns or anchovy essence if using. Then, gently stir in the fish.
* Place the fish and sauce in a suitable ovenproof dish. Spread the mashed potato on top and make a criss-cross pattern with the prongs of a fork.
* Bake in the oven for 20–25 minutes until the potato is beginning to brown. Brown a little more under a pre-heated grill if you like.

SMOKY FISH PIE
....

SERVES 4

1 onion, chopped
2 cloves garlic, peeled and finely chopped
1 × 14-oz (400-g) tin tomatoes
pinch of mixed dried herbs
salt and freshly milled black pepper
8 oz (225 g) cod or other white fish, cooked and flaked
8 oz (225 g) smoked cod or smoked haddock, cooked and flaked
chopped fresh parsley
1 lb (450 g) potatoes, boiled in their jackets
2 oz (50 g) Edam cheese, grated

* Pre-heat the oven to gas mark 4, 350°F (180°C).
* 'Dry fry' (see p. 86) the onion and garlic in a large pan, add the tomatoes and herbs and simmer until sauce thickens, season to taste.
* Put the flaked fish and sauce into an ovenproof dish, mix in the chopped parsley. Peel the cooked potatoes and cut them into thin slices. Place them, overlapping, on top of the fish mixture.
* Sprinkle the top of the pie with grated cheese. Bake in the oven until golden brown.

CRUNCHY FISH BAKE

SERVES 4

1 lb (450 g) cod or haddock fillets
4 oz (100 g) mushrooms, thinly sliced
½ onion, finely chopped
juice of 1 lemon
salt and freshly milled black pepper
pinch of mixed dried herbs
2 slices wholemeal bread, toasted and crumbed

❋ Pre-heat the oven to gas mark 4, 350°F (180°C).

❋ Divide the fish into portions and place in the bottom of a shallow casserole. Cover with the mushrooms and onions and pour in the lemon juice.

❋ Season to taste, sprinkle over the herbs and cover with foil. Bake for 30 minutes.

❋ Remove the foil. Sprinkle the toasted crumbs over the top. Return to the oven for a further 10 minutes. Serve.

CHINESE FISH AND NOODLES

SERVES 1

This recipe could be cooked in a microwave if you prefer. You would have to consult your microwave manual for accurate timings, but it should take about 5–7 minutes. Remember, do not use foil in the microwave – use greaseproof paper.

6 oz (175 g) boneless and skinless haddock fillet or any other white fish, fresh or frozen
1 carrot, peeled and cut into matchsticks
3 spring onions, shredded
1 clove garlic, peeled and finely chopped
1 teaspoon peeled and finely chopped fresh root ginger
1 tablespoon soy sauce

1 tablespoon dry sherry or dry vermouth
3 oz (75 g) Chinese noodles (preferably wholewheat)

- Pre-heat the oven to gas mark 6, 400°F (200°C).
- Cut a piece of foil or greaseproof paper big enough to make an envelope for the fish.
- Place the fish on the foil or paper and sprinkle the carrot, onions, garlic and ginger on top. Combine the soy sauce with the sherry or vermouth and pour on. Fold up the parcel and turn over all the edges several times to make a tight seal.
- Cook in the oven for 10–15 minutes (if fish is frozen for 20–25 minutes). Serve with the noodles, cooked as directed on the packet.

SARDINE FISHCAKES

SERVES 1
8 oz (225 g) potatoes
1 tin sardines, in brine
1 tablespoon chopped fresh parsley (optional)
salt and freshly milled black pepper
squeeze of lemon

- Peel the potatoes and simmer until tender. Drain and mash thoroughly.
- Drain the sardines and stir into the potatoes with the parsley if you are using it. Season with salt, pepper and lemon juice. Shape into 2 fishcakes using floured hands. 'Dry fry' (see p. 86) or grill on a lightly oiled sheet of aluminium foil for 2–3 minutes on each side or until beginning to brown.

STUFFED SARDINES

SERVES 2

4 large or 6 medium-sized sardines fresh or frozen and thawed
1 clove garlic, peeled and finely chopped
1½ oz (40 g) wholemeal breadcrumbs
1 tablespoon finely chopped fresh parsley
1 tablespoon finely chopped sorrel or spinach
zest and juice of ½ lemon
salt and freshly milled black pepper

* Pre-heat the oven to gas mark 6, 400°F (200°C).
* Cut the head and tail off each fish. Slit down the stomach and clean. Place skin side up and run your finger down the backbone, pressing firmly. You should find that the backbone and adjoining bones can now be removed. If other small bones remain, remove them.
* Mix together the garlic, breadcrumbs, parsley, sorrel or spinach (if using) and the juice and finely chopped zest of the lemon. Season and stuff the sardines with this mixture and reshape.
* Place the sardines side-by-side on a large piece of foil and fold over foil to make a parcel, sealing the edges securely. Cook in the oven for 25 minutes.
* Serve with the other half of the lemon.

TOMATO AND SARDINE PIZZA
··

Easy-blend yeast is quick and easy to use.

SERVES 1
A good pinch of salt
1 scant flat teaspoon easy-blend yeast
3 oz (75 g) strong plain white flour
warm water to mix
3 ripe tomatoes or 7-oz (200-g) tin chopped tomatoes, drained
½ teaspoon dried or 1 tablespoon chopped fresh oregano
1 clove garlic, peeled and finely chopped (optional)
2 oz (50 g) mushrooms, sliced
1 tin sardines in brine, drained
salt and freshly milled black pepper

✳ Pre-heat the oven to gas mark 6, 400°F (200°C).

✳ Mix the salt and yeast with the flour and add just enough hand-hot water to blend into a workable dough (this takes 10–15 seconds in a food processor). Knead the dough between the floured palms of your hands for 2 or 3 minutes or process for another minute or so. Put the dough in a floured polythene bag and leave in a warm place while you prepare the vegetables. Try to leave it for 15–20 minutes.

✳ If you are using fresh tomatoes, peel and chop them and leave them to drain in a sieve. Mix the oregano and garlic, plus salt and freshly milled black pepper, into the chopped tomatoes or the drained tinned tomatoes.

✳ Roll or press out the dough to about a 10-inch (25-cm) round. Place it on a very lightly oiled baking sheet or piece of aluminium foil.

✳ Arrange the sliced mushrooms over the pizza and then evenly distribute the tomato mixture on top. Arrange the sardines on top of this.

✳ Bake for about 25 minutes until the dough is cooked and the edges are crisp and browning.

TUNA OMELETTE

SERVES 1

1 clove garlic, peeled and finely chopped
2 oz (50 g) tuna in brine or water, drained and flaked
1 tablespoon 8% fromage frais or Greek yoghurt (see p. 90)
1 tablespoon finely chopped fresh parsley
salt and freshly milled black pepper
2 eggs (see p. 89)
1 tablespoon skimmed milk

❋ 'Dry fry' (see p. 86) the garlic in a heavy non-stick frying-pan until soft but not coloured. Add the tuna and warm through. Take off the heat and add the fromage frais or yoghurt and the parsley. Stir well, season and keep warm but be very careful not to bring to boiling point.

❋ Lightly whisk the eggs and add the milk and some seasoning.

❋ Heat another heavy non-stick frying-pan – about 7–8 inches (18–20 cm) across – on a medium heat. When it is hot, add the eggs and stir 2 or 3 times with a wooden spoon, bringing the setting eggs from the edge to the centre and allowing the liquid egg to flow onto the pan's surface. Leave for a minute or so until the omelette is set but is still moist on top.

❋ Distribute the hot filling across the centre of the omelette; fold the omelette and turn out of the pan onto a hot plate.

TUNA AND MUSHROOM SUPREME

SERVES 1

½ small onion, finely chopped
1 clove garlic, peeled and finely chopped (optional)
2 oz (50 g) mushrooms, wiped and chopped
3 oz (75 g) tuna in brine or water, drained
1–2 teaspoons lemon juice

1 quantity of White sauce (see p. 345)
salt and freshly milled black pepper
chopped fresh parsley to garnish

* 'Dry fry' (see p. 86) the onion and garlic (if using) until very soft but don't allow them to colour. Add the mushrooms and continue to stir and fry for 1–2 minutes until the juices being to run.

* Stir this onion and mushroom mixture with the tuna and lemon juice into the White sauce, stir, and cook gently until heated right through.

* Season and serve sprinkled with parsley.

TUNA CASSOULET

SERVES 2
1 oz (25 g) wholemeal breadcrumbs
½ oz (15 g) freshly grated Parmesan cheese
1 × 7-oz (200-g) tin tuna in brine or water, drained
1 × 14-oz (400-g) tin white kidney beans (cannellini beans)
½ oz (15 g) onion, finely chopped
1 clove garlic, peeled and finely chopped (optional)
7-oz (200-g) tin chopped tomatoes or 3 fresh tomatoes, skinned
and chopped and 1 tablespoon tomato purée mixed with 1
tablespoon of water

* Pre-heat the oven to gas mark 6, 400°F (200°C).

* Mix together the breadcrumbs and cheese. Combine and mix well all the other ingredients and place in an ovenproof casserole.

* Top with the breadcrumb and cheese mixture and bake in the oven for 40–45 minutes until the top is browned.

TUNA AND BULGAR RISOTTO

You could make this dish using brown rice; you will need to keep adding a little water until the rice is cooked, which will take about 40 minutes. If you're really hungry you could use 3 oz (75 g) of bulgar wheat or rice per person without increasing the calories too much – and that's much better than being tempted to snack or have something sugary later. Another alternative is to use chopped cooked chicken instead of tuna: about 6 oz (175 g). In this case, you could use chicken stock instead of water.

SERVES 2
1 onion, finely chopped
1 clove garlic, peeled and finely chopped
4 oz (100 g) bulgar wheat (burghul, pourgouri, or cracked wheat)
2 oz (50 g) frozen peas
1 × 7-oz (200-g) tin tuna in brine or water, drained
salt and freshly milled black pepper
½ oz (15 g) Edam cheese, grated

* 'Dry fry' (see p. 86) the onion and garlic in a heavy non-stick frying-pan. Add the bulgar wheat and fry gently for a further couple of minutes.
* Add 2 cups of water and stir well. Simmer gently until most of the water has been absorbed.
* Add the peas and tuna and stir until all is hot. Season with salt and pepper.
* Serve on heated plates and sprinkle with the grated cheese.

TUNA PASTA RIBBONS

SERVES 4

1 × 14-oz (400-g) tin tomatoes
4 oz (100 g) mushrooms, sliced
½–1 green or red pepper, de-seeded and chopped
½ onion, chopped
2 teaspoons tomato purée
1 clove garlic, peeled and crushed
1 × 7-oz (200-g) tin tuna, in brine or water, drained
dried or chopped fresh oregano to taste
salt and freshly milled black pepper
8 oz (225 g) dried tagliatelle

✳ Simmer together the tinned tomatoes, mushrooms, peppers, onion, tomato purée and garlic until the vegetables are soft.

✳ Meanwhile boil the pasta in lightly salted water until it is cooked but still firm. Drain.

✳ Add the tuna to the tomato mixture together with the oregano and season to taste. Then add the cooked tagliatelle and mix well. Serve.

PRAWN AND FENNEL RISOTTO

For this tasty risotto, the ideal rice to use is Arborio or Italian risotto rice. It's available in many supermarkets these days but, otherwise, pudding rice will do.

SERVES 1

1 × 4 oz (100 g) head Florence fennel
½ onion, finely chopped
1 clove garlic, peeled and finely chopped (optional)
2 oz (50 g) white round rice (preferably Arborio or Italian risotto
salt and freshly milled black pepper
2 oz (50 g) prawns, fresh or frozen and thawed
½ tablespoon freshly grated Parmesan cheese

❋ Finely chop the fennel and reserve some leaves for garnishing later.

❋ 'Dry fry' (see p. 86) the onion and garlic until soft, add the fennel and stir and fry for another couple of minutes. Add the rice and stir thoroughly.

❋ Add hot water, a cupful at a time and simmer (see method on p. 260). When the rice is cooked, season, add the prawns, stir and warm thoroughly but do not overheat.

❋ Serve sprinkled with the Parmesan and reserved fennel leaves.

PASTA SHELLS WITH PRAWNS, LIME AND DILL

This is a delectable pasta dish and very quick to make. You can use ½ lemon instead of the lime but it's not as good!

SERVES 1

3½ oz (90 g) pasta shells or other pasta shapes
½ clove garlic, peeled and finely chopped
juice and finely grated zest of ½ lime (or lemon)
3 oz (75 g) prawns, fresh or frozen and thawed
2 tablespoons Greek yoghurt
1 tablespoon skimmed milk
salt and freshly milled black pepper
1 tablespoon finely chopped fresh dill
1 tablespoon freshly grated Parmesan cheese

* Cook the pasta in salted boiling water for 10–12 minutes until it's tender but still has 'a bite'.
* Meanwhile, heat the garlic with the lime juice and zest. Add the prawns and heat them gently: remember they're already cooked so if you cook them again, they'll go rubbery.
* When the pasta is nearly ready, whisk together the yoghurt and milk and add to the lime and prawn mixture. Heat thoroughly but DO NOT BOIL. Season to taste.
* Drain the pasta, mix thoroughly with the sauce and stir in the dill.
* Serve on a heated plate, sprinkled with the grated Parmesan cheese.

MONKFISH PROVENÇALE

Here's a taste of the Mediterranean. You could use a steak of cod or haddock or any other white fish if you prefer.

SERVES 1

4 oz (100 g) monkfish
½ onion, finely chopped
1–2 cloves garlic, peeled and finely chopped
3 ripe medium tomatoes, peeled and chopped or 1 × 7-oz (200-g)
tin chopped tomatoes
1½ oz (40 g) black olives, unstoned
1 tablespoon finely chopped fresh basil or 1 tablespoon finely
chopped fresh oregano
salt and freshly milled black pepper
squeeze of lemon juice

* Cut the monkfish into 1½-inch (4-cm) chunks.
* 'Dry fry' (see p. 86) the onion and garlic until soft, add the tomatoes and simmer for 10 minutes until reduced a little.
* Add the monkfish to the sauce and simmer for just 2–3 minutes until it is white and opaque. (If you are using cod or haddock steaks, simmer for 2 or 3 minutes longer or until cooked.) Add the olives towards the end of the cooking time and heat through.
* Stir in the herbs and season with salt and freshly milled black pepper and a squeeze of lemon juice.

KEDGEREE
....

*This is adapted from the famous Anglo-Indian dish which was a
favourite for breakfast during the days of the Raj.*

SERVES 1

5 oz (150 g) smoked haddock
1 small onion, finely chopped
3 oz (75 g) long-grain brown rice
1–2 teaspoons curry powder
salt and freshly milled black pepper
juice of ½ lemon
1 tablespoon finely chopped fresh parsley
2 tablespoons low-fat natural yoghurt

✳ Poach the haddock in enough water to cover it. Then drain
and reserve the cooking liquid. Flake the haddock when it's
cool.

✳ 'Dry fry' (see p. 86) the onion until soft, add the rice and
stir and fry for a few seconds more. Sprinkle on the curry
powder and stir and fry for another minute.

✳ Mix in the cooking liquid from the fish and start to simmer.
Simmer until the rice is tender (about 25–30 minutes)
adding more water as necessary. Stir frequently.

✳ When the rice is cooked, gently stir in the flaked haddock
and season with salt, freshly milled black pepper and the
lemon juice. Heat everything through thoroughly. Take off
the heat and stir in the parsley and yoghurt, mix well and
serve.

POULTRY

CHICKEN IN BARBECUE SAUCE

SERVES 1

1 teaspoon tomato purée mixed with 2 teaspoons of water or
1 tablespoon tomato ketchup
1 tablespoon soy sauce
1 tablespoon wine or *cider vinegar*
1 tablespoon sherry or *vermouth*
½ teaspoon sugar
1 clove garlic, peeled and sliced
4–5 oz (100–150 g) boneless, skinless chicken breast
½ teaspoon polyunsaturated oil (e.g. sunflower)

✻ Whisk together the first 5 ingredients. Add the sliced garlic.

✻ Place the chicken in a dish, pour over the sauce and cover and marinate in the fridge for at least 6 and up to 24 hours.

✻ Next, remove the chicken and place on a piece of foil lightly brushed with the polyunsaturated oil (see p. 87). The foil should be large enough to make a closed parcel over the chicken.

✻ Spoon over the sauce and close up the foil, sealing the joins by folding over several times.

✻ Bake at gas mark 4, 350°F (180°C) for 20 minutes. Then open the foil and bake for a further 10 minutes until the chicken begins to brown slightly.

✻ Serve the chicken, spooning any remaining sauce.

MARINATED AND DEVILLED CHICKEN

SERVES 1

7–8 oz (200–225 g) chicken drumsticks or thighs (weight
including bone), skin removed
2 cloves garlic, peeled and crushed
salt and freshly milled black pepper
juice of ½ lemon

✳ Make 3 or 4 slashes through to the bone with a sharp knife
on each side of the chicken pieces.

✳ Place the chicken in a shallow dish and smear the crushed
garlic over both sides of the pieces. Grind plenty (or to taste)
of black pepper over both sides of the chicken and then
pour over the lemon juice.

✳ Cover the dish and leave the chicken to marinate in the
fridge for at least 6 and up to 24 hours. Turn often.

✳ Drain the chicken and scrape off the garlic.

✳ Heat the grill to its highest setting and grill the chicken for
15–20 minutes, turning frequently until it begins to char
slightly and the juice runs clear when a knife is inserted. Do
not overcook though – the idea is that it is still moist inside.

✳ Sprinkle a little salt on the chicken, some more black pepper
and perhaps another squeeze of lemon and serve.

GRILLED CHICKEN ROSEMARY

SERVES 1

1 × 8-oz (225-g) chicken joint, skinned
juice of 1 lemon
pinch of fresh or dried rosemary
freshly milled black pepper

✳ Score the top of the chicken joint with a sharp knife and rub
with lemon juice, rosemary and black pepper.

✳ Grill for about 15 minutes each side.

CHICKEN PROVENÇALE
....

Wholemeal breadcrumbs can be made instantly in a food processor. If you don't have one, you can grate bread which is a couple of days old or toast the bread, cool, place in a polythene bag and bash with a rolling pin. In this case, add the topping halfway through cooking.

For a variation, add 1 finely chopped red or green pepper with the onions and garlic when making the tomato sauce.

SERVES 4

1 quantity of Tomato sauce (see p. 258)
4 × 5-oz (150-g) boneless and skinless chicken breasts, fresh or frozen and thawed
1 oz (25 g) freshly grated Parmesan cheese
1 oz (25 g) wholemeal breadcrumbs

❋ Pre-heat the oven to gas mark 6, 400°F (200°C).
❋ Place 2 tablespoons of the Tomato sauce on the bottom of an ovenproof dish. Arrange the chicken on top and pour over the rest of the Tomato sauce. Mix the cheese and breadcrumbs together and sprinkle on top of the sauce.
❋ Bake in the oven for 25–30 minutes, until browned.

CHICKEN STIR-FRY
....

SERVES 1

4–5 oz (100–150 g) boneless, skinless chicken breast
4–5 spring onions, thickly sliced
1 clove garlic, peeled and finely chopped
1 red, green or yellow pepper, de-seeded and sliced
1 tablespoon soy sauce
1 tablespoon tomato ketchup or tomato purée
1–2 tablespoons wine or cider vinegar

* Slice the chicken into thin, bite-size pieces.
* 'Dry fry' (see p. 86) the white part of the onions and the garlic for 1–2 minutes.
* Add the sliced chicken and stir-fry for 2–3 minutes.
* Add the de-seeded, sliced pepper and continue to stir-fry for another 2–3 minutes or until the chicken is cooked. If things begin to stick, add a tablespoon of water.
* Mix the soy sauce, tomato ketchup (or purée) and the vinegar together and add to the chicken mixture, stirring well.
* Mix the sliced green part of the spring onions in and serve.

SPICY CHICKEN WITH APPLE

SERVES 1

½ small onion, chopped
1–2 teaspoons mild curry powder
7 fl oz (200 ml) Chicken stock (see p. 348)
4 oz (100 g) cauliflower, chopped
4 oz (100 g) cooking apple, peeled and chopped
1 teaspoon lemon juice
1 teaspoon tomato purée
8 oz (225 g) boneless chicken breast, skinned and sliced
salt and freshly milled black pepper

* 'Dry fry' (see p. 86) the onion until soft. Add the curry powder and stir well for a minute or so.
* Add the stock, cauliflower, apple, lemon juice, tomato purée and chicken breast and simmer for 25–30 minutes.
* Season and serve with brown rice.

OVENBAKED CRISPY CHICKEN

*This is a very quick and simple dish. Make the breadcrumbs in a
liquidiser or food processor or, if using 1- or 2-day-old bread, on a
grater.*

SERVES 1

1½ tablespoons wholemeal breadcrumbs
½ tablespoon grated Parmesan or low-fat Cheddar cheese
½ teaspoon finely grated lemon zest (optional)
salt and freshly milled black pepper
2 teaspoons low-fat natural yoghurt
2 teaspoons skimmed milk
4–5 oz (100–150 g) skinless, boneless chicken breast or 6–7 oz
(175–200 g) skinless chicken breast on the bone

- ❋ Pre-heat the oven to gas mark 4, 350°F (180°C).
- ❋ Mix together the breadcrumbs, cheese, lemon zest (if using),
  season and place in a shallow dish or on a plate.
- ❋ Mix together the yoghurt and milk and dip the chicken into
  this or spread it all over it.
- ❋ Turn the chicken several times in the breadcrumb mixture,
  pressing the mixture on so that chicken is coated all over.
- ❋ Bake the chicken on a very lightly oiled oven tray or piece
  of baking foil, uncovered, in the oven for 25–35 minutes
  until the chicken is cooked and the coating is brown and
  crispy.

CHICKEN CURRY

Serve this with the Fresh tomato and onion chutney on p. 344. This is a mild, chicken Korma-type curry. If you prefer, you can use 1–2 teaspoons of mild curry powder in place of the individual spices.

SERVES 1

4-5 oz (100-150 g) boneless, skinless chicken breast
½ small onion, finely chopped
1 clove garlic, peeled and finely chopped
1 × 1-inch (2.6-cm) piece fresh root ginger, peeled and finely chopped
1 teaspoon ground coriander
½ teaspoon turmeric
4–5 cardamom pods
5 fl oz (150 ml) Chicken stock (see p. 348)
salt and freshly milled black pepper
squeeze of lemon juice
1 tablespoon Greek yoghurt or 8% fromage frais (see p. 90)

❋ Cut the chicken into large cubes.
❋ 'Dry fry' (see p. 86) the onion, garlic and ginger for 2–3 minutes.
❋ Add all the spices and fry for 1 minute.
❋ Add the chicken and fry for 2 minutes, stirring all the time, and adding a tablespoon of water if it begins to stick.
❋ Now pour in the Chicken stock, stir well, and simmer gently for 12–15 minutes until the chicken is cooked.
❋ Season with salt, freshly milled black pepper and lemon juice and, off the heat, stir in the yoghurt or fromage frais and mix well.

ROAST CHICKEN WITH MUSHROOMS

This recipe you can serve to your family and they won't know it's a 'slimming dish'. The creamy mushroom sauce only provides a couple of tablespoons each – but any lack of quantity is made up for in the taste.

This, incidentally, is a way of roasting chicken without adding any fat at all. I now always roast a chicken in this way – in spite of nearly every cookery book I've ever read which tells you chicken is dry if you don't add extra fat. I think the truth is that chicken is dry if you overcook it. The traditional roasting formula is '20 minutes a pound and 20 over for good luck!'. However, I find that for a 3-lb (1.5-kg) chicken, an hour at gas mark 6, 400°F, (200°C) is about right. Oven temperatures vary from oven to oven so any suggested roasting time can only be approximate.

Obviously, I'm not suggesting that you eat your chicken rare – that may be dangerous – but chicken is cooked and safe well before it becomes dry. If you're unsure, you can check for 'doneness' by piercing the thigh with a knife or skewer (the juices should be clear and yellow, not pink) or by tugging at the leg (it should be easy to pull it away from the body).

SERVES 4

1 × 3-lb (1.5-kg) chicken
3 cloves garlic, peeled and flattened with the side of a knife
½ lemon
8 oz (225 g) large open flat mushrooms, wiped and roughly chopped
10 fl oz (300 ml) Chicken stock (see p. 348)
2 tablespoons dry white wine or dry white vermouth (optional)
3 tablespoons 8% fromage frais or Greek yoghurt (see p. 90)
salt and freshly milled black pepper

* Pre-heat the oven to gas mark 6, 400°F (200°C).
* Try to use a heavy non-stick roasting tin (and also, if you have one, a roasting rack). Prepare the chicken by discarding

the lump of fat which is just inside the body cavity from the parson's nose. Place the garlic and lemon in the body cavity.

❋ Roast the chicken, breast upwards, for about an hour (see notes above).

❋ Remove the chicken to a heated plate, tipping the juices from the body cavity into the roasting tin. Let the chicken rest in a warm place.

❋ Let the juices in the roasting tin cool for a minute or so. Then tip up to one side and carefully spoon off all the fat floating on top and discard. Take your time over this: try to leave less than 1 tablespoon of fat, but leave as much as possible of the brown tasty residue.

❋ Now put the roasting tin over a gentle heat and fry the mushrooms in the residue for 1–2 minutes, adding a tablespoon of water if they stick.

❋ Add the stock and wine (if using) and use a wooden spoon to scrape up all the residue. Reduce (either in the tin or having poured everything into a sturdier pan) by at least half.

❋ Remove from the heat, whisk in the fromage frais or Greek yoghurt and season. Serve with the chicken.

❋ Remove the chicken skin and serve a portion of breast for yourself.

ROAST CHICKEN WITH FRESH HERBS

The recipe is really very simple. Even if the only fresh herb you can lay your hands on is parsley, it's worth making this recipe.

SERVES 4
1 × 3-lb (1.5-kg) chicken
1 tablespoon chopped fresh parsley, chives, tarragon and chervil
½ clove garlic, peeled and very finely chopped
2 tablespoons 8% fromage frais (see p. 90)
salt and freshly milled black pepper
10 fl oz (300 ml) Chicken stock (see p. 348)

❋ Pre-heat the oven to gas mark 6, 400°F (200°C).

❋ Mix the herbs and garlic into the fromage frais and stir well. Season lightly.

❋ Prepare the chicken by discarding the lump of fat which is just inside the body cavity from the parson's nose. Now turn the chicken round and, beginning at the neck, work your fingers into the gap between the skin and the breast. Be careful not to break the skin and gently work your whole hand in over the breast and across to each leg, breaking down the adhesions with a finger as you go. This is much easier to do than it sounds and not at all unpleasant.

❋ Now work the fromage frais mixture, between the skin and the flesh, right up over the breast and over each leg, using your fingers or a spoon.

❋ Roast the chicken for about an hour (see note about roasting chickens on p. 298). You should be aware that the fromage frais makes the skin brown sooner and more deeply than usual, so don't be misled by this and if necessary protect the top of the chicken with a small square of foil.

❋ Remove the chicken to a heated plate, tipping the juices from the cavity back into the roasting tin. Let the chicken rest in a warm place.

❋ Let the juices in the roasting tin cool for a minute or so, then tip up one side and carefully spoon off all the fat floating on top and discard. Try to leave less than 1 tablespoon of fat but, of course, as much of the bottom brown residue as possible.

❊ Add the chicken stock, scrape up all the residue with a wooden spoon, and reduce the stock by about half. Season.

❊ Serve the chicken cut into portions rather than carved. Cut into 2 drumsticks, 2 thighs, and the breast cut into 4. Serve yourself 2 breast portions, with the skin removed. Pour over the sauce.

CHICKEN AND VEGETABLE RICE

Useful for left-over brown rice and left-over chicken.

SERVES 1
½ small onion, chopped
¼ green pepper, de-seeded and chopped
2 oz (50 g) peas
4 oz (100 g) cooked brown rice
½ teaspoon dried mixed herbs or ½ tablespoon chopped fresh
oregano
½ teaspoon dried oregano or ½ tablespoon chopped fresh mixed
herbs
1 × 7-oz (200-g) tin tomatoes
salt and freshly milled black pepper
2 oz (50 g) cold cooked chicken, diced
2 oz (50 g) mushrooms, chopped

❊ 'Dry fry' (see p. 86) the onion until soft. Add the green pepper, peas and rice and fry for a further minute.

❊ Add the herbs and tomatoes and season well and simmer for 2 minutes.

❊ Add the chicken and mushrooms. Warm through thoroughly and serve.

TURKEY 'SALTIMBOCCA'

The original Roman version of this (which literally means 'jump in the mouth') uses veal, but turkey or chicken works well.

SERVES 1

4–5 oz (100–150 g) skinless, boneless turkey or chicken breast
2 very thin slices of Parma ham
3 fresh sage leaves
2 tablespoons Marsala or medium sherry
1 tablespoon water
salt and freshly milled black pepper
squeeze of lemon juice

* Slice the turkey or chicken horizontally into 3 escalopes. Beat each one with a rolling pin between 2 sheets of greaseproof paper until it has increased in size by at least half as much again.
* Cut the fat from the ham and arrange pieces of the ham evenly over the escalopes. Break each sage leaf in half and place on the escalopes.
* Now roll each escalope up and secure with half a wooden cocktail stick or toothpick.
* 'Dry fry' (see p. 86) the little rolls for 10–12 minutes or until the turkey is cooked. Remove and keep them warm.
* Pour the Marsala (or sherry) and the water into the pan and let it bubble and reduce to about half, scraping up any residue on the bottom of the pan with a wooden spoon. Taste and season with salt, pepper and lemon juice.
* Pour the syrupy sauce around the rolls and serve.

TURKEY ESCALOPES MARSALA

This Italian dish is extremely quick to make. You can use chicken instead of turkey.

SERVES 1

4–5 oz (100–150 g) skinless, boneless turkey breast fillet
2 tablespoons Marsala or medium sherry
2 tablespoons water or Chicken stock (see p. 348)
salt and freshly milled black pepper
squeeze of lemon juice
chopped parsley to garnish (optional)

* Slice the turkey horizontally into 2 or 3 escalopes. Beat them with a rolling pin between 2 sheets of greaseproof paper until they have increased in size by about half as much again.
* Heat a heavy non-stick frying-pan and quickly 'dry fry' (see p. 86) the turkey escalopes on both sides until they are just cooked (2–3 minutes). Remove from the pan and keep warm.
* Pour into the pan the Marsala (or sherry) and stock (or water). Boil fiercely for a minute or two, stirring and scraping up and incorporating any turkey residue in the pan. Reduce the sauce by about half.
* Taste and season with salt, pepper and lemon juice.
* Pour over the turkey escalopes and sprinkle with chopped parsley if wished.

TURKEY KEBABS MARINATED IN YOGHURT, LIME AND GINGER

These kebabs taste wonderful and are something I choose to serve to friends for pleasure – not slimming!

SERVES 1

4–5 oz (100–150 g) skinless, boneless turkey breast fillets
3 tablespoons low-fat natural yoghurt
zest and juice of ½ lime or lemon
1 clove garlic, peeled and sliced
1 × 1-inch (2.5-cm) piece fresh root ginger, peeled and sliced

* Cut the turkey into even pieces of about 1½ inches (4 cm).
* Put the yoghurt into a bowl big enough to hold the turkey and whisk it lightly. Mix in the lime zest and juice, the garlic and the ginger.
* Turn the turkey pieces in the yoghurt mixture, cover and marinate in the fridge for at least 6 and up to 24 hours.
* Drain the turkey pieces from the yoghurt marinade and discard the marinade. Thread the turkey on a metal skewer.
* Heat the grill to its highest setting. Grill the kebabs for 8–10 minutes turning frequently. The edges will just be going brown and the meat will be white all the way through: don't overcook or they will be dry.
* Serve, with a squeeze of lime or lemon juice if you like.

TURKEYBALLS IN MUSHROOM AND YOGHURT SAUCE

SERVES 1

½ small onion
1 clove garlic, peeled
4 oz (100 g) skinless, boneless turkey or chicken breast
3 oz (75 g) mushrooms
1 oz (25 g) wholemeal breadcrumbs
salt and freshly milled black pepper
3 tablespoons low-fat natural yoghurt
squeeze of lemon juice

* Process the onion and garlic in a food processor until finely minced. Add the turkey (or chicken) and 1 oz (25 g) of the mushrooms and process for 1–2 minutes until the meat is very finely chopped.

* Add the breadcrumbs and seasoning. Process briefly to mix.

* Divide the mixture into 6 equal portions, wet your hands, and roll each portion into a ball between your palms.

* 'Dry fry' (see p. 86) the balls for 6–7 minutes over a medium heat until they are browning on the outside and cooked inside. Remove the balls from the pan and keep warm.

* Slice the remaining mushrooms and 'dry fry' for about 2 minutes until their juices begin to run. Add a tablespoon or so of water and stir vigorously with a wooden spoon to release any residue on the bottom of the pan. When the water has almost evaporated, remove the pan from the heat and stir in the yoghurt. Mix well and season with salt, freshly milled black pepper and lemon juice.

* Serve the sauce with the turkeyballs.

NOTE You could also use left-over cooked chicken or turkey instead.

TURKEY BURGERS
....

Turkey breast meat is extremely low in fat – you can also use chicken breast which is almost as low in fat. These turkey burgers are easy to make but you do need a food processor to gain the right texture so they stick together. Make the breadcrumbs separately beforehand in the food processor.

SERVES 1

½ small onion
1 clove garlic, peeled
4 oz (100 g) skinless, boneless turkey or chicken breast
1 oz (25 g) wholemeal breadcrumbs
1 tablespoon finely chopped parsley or tarragon
salt and freshly milled black pepper

❋ Process the onion and garlic until finely minced. Add the turkey or chicken and process 1–2 minutes until the meat is very finely chopped.

❋ Add the breadcrumbs, parsley (or tarragon) and seasoning and process briefly to mix.

❋ Using your hands, shape the mixture and press into 2 burger shapes.

❋ Grill fiercely for 7–8 minutes, turning once, until the outside is crisp and brown and the inside cooked but still moist.

❋ Alternatively, 'dry fry' (see p. 86) in a heavy non-stick frying-pan for the same length of time.

NOTE These can also be made using cooked left-over chicken or turkey. In this case, add a teaspoon or two of low-fat natural yoghurt to keep them moist and don't overcook.

MEAT

PORK ESCALOPES WITH WHITE WINE

This is a very simple and quick recipe but it tastes delicious.

SERVES 1

4–5 oz (100-150 g) pork tenderloin or fillet (in 3 or 4 slices)
1–2 cloves garlic, peeled and halved
5 tablespoons dry white wine or vermouth
salt and freshly milled black pepper
chopped parsley to garnish (optional)

✳ Trim off any visible fat and put the slices of pork between 2 sheets of greaseproof paper and beat them gently with the end of a rolling pin until they have increased in size by about half as much again.

✳ 'Dry fry' (see p. 86) the garlic in a heavy non-stick frying-pan for 1–2 minutes.

✳ Push the garlic to one side and turn up the heat. Quickly fry the pork for about 1½ minutes on each side until cooked through. Don't overcook.

✳ Remove the pork to a heated plate and keep warm. Discard the garlic.

✳ Pour the wine into the pan and let it boil rapidly, scraping into it with a wooden spoon any residue on the pan from the pork. Boil until reduced by half. Season.

✳ Pour the sauce over the pork and sprinkle with chopped parsley if you like.

QUICK STIR-FRIED PORK WITH BEANSPROUTS

SERVES 1

4 oz (100 g) pork fillet or tenderloin or boneless steak
½ onion, finely sliced
1 clove garlic, peeled and finely chopped
1 x 1-inch (2.5-cm) piece fresh root ginger, peeled and finely chopped
½ red or green pepper, de-seeded and sliced
4 oz (100 g) beansprouts
1 tablespoon black bean sauce or yellow bean sauce or soy sauce
1 tablespoon dry sherry or white wine or vermouth

※ Trim all fat from the pork and slice the meat into very thin, bite-size pieces.
※ 'Dry fry' (see p. 86) the onion, garlic and ginger for a minute or so. Add the pork and pepper and continue to stir and fry for 5–6 minutes (adding a tablespoon of water if they start to stick) until the pork is cooked.
※ Add the beansprouts, mix thoroughly and heat for 1 minute so they are hot but still crisp. Mix whichever sauce you have chosen with the sherry or wine, add to the pan, mixing well.
※ Bring to the boil for 10–20 seconds and serve immediately.

QUICK SWEET AND SOUR PORK

SERVES 1

4 oz (100 g) pork fillet or tenderloin or boneless steak
½ onion, thickly sliced
½ red or green pepper, de-seeded and thickly sliced
1 ring pineapple, tinned in natural juices, drained or 10 pineapple chunks, tinned in natural juice, drained
1 tablespoon pineapple juice (from tin)
1 tablespoon tomato ketchup or tomato purée

1 tablespoon soy sauce
1–2 teaspoons wine or cider vinegar
¼ teaspoon cornflour

❋ Trim all fat off the pork and cut the meat into thin, bite-size pieces.

❋ 'Dry fry' (see p. 86) the pork, onion and pepper for 5–6 minutes until the pork is cooked and the vegetables are still slightly crunchy. Add the pineapple and warm through.

❋ Whisk together all the other ingredients. Add to the pan, bring to the boil and simmer for a couple of minutes. Serve immediately.

VEAL AL LIMONE

If you prefer you could make this using turkey instead.

SERVES 2
2 × 3–4 oz (75–100 g) veal escalopes
juice of ½ large lemon
4 tablespoons dry vermouth or dry white wine
salt and freshly milled black pepper
sprigs of parsley to garnish

❋ Place the veal escalopes between sheets of greaseproof paper and beat with a steak mallet or a rolling pin until the veal is very thin.

❋ 'Dry fry' (see p. 86) the veal in a heavy non-stick frying-pan. Be careful not to overcook it. Remove and keep warm.

❋ Add the lemon juice and the vermouth to the pan. Stir with a wooden spoon to incorporate the juices of the veal. Boil rapidly for about 1 minute, season, pour over the veal and serve, garnished with the parsley.

CALF'S OR LAMB'S LIVER WITH ORANGE AND VERMOUTH

....

I think calf's liver is more delicious, but it is more expensive.

SERVES 1
1 clove garlic, peeled and sliced
3½–4 oz (90–100 g) calf's or lamb's liver in thin, even slices
2 tablespoons dry white vermouth
2 tablespoons orange juice
salt and freshly milled black pepper
parsley to garnish

* 'Dry fry' (see p. 86) the slices of garlic for 1 or 2 minutes in a heavy non-stick frying-pan.
* Push the garlic to one side, turn up the heat slightly, and quickly fry the liver for about 45 seconds–1 minute on each side. It should be just cooked through and still slightly pink. If you prefer it a bit more done, cook for another 30 seconds or so on each side but don't overcook it.
* Place the liver on a heated plate and keep warm but not hot. Discard the garlic.
* Put the vermouth and orange juice in the frying-pan, turn up the heat, and stir to dislodge any stuck-on residue from the garlic or liver (the tasty bits!). Boil the mixture until it is reduced by half. Season to taste.
* Pour over the liver and serve garnished with parsley.

BEEF AND VEGETABLE CURRY

SERVES 4

1 medium onion, chopped
1 lb (450 g) lean stewing beef, trimmed of all fat and cut into cubes
8 oz (225 g) cooking apples, peeled and chopped
1 × 14-oz (400-g) tin tomatoes
10 fl oz (300 ml) beef stock
salt and freshly milled black pepper
2–3 teaspoons mild curry powder or 1–2 hot or to taste

- 'Dry fry' (see p. 86) the onions until soft. Add the beef, sprinkle with curry powder and continue to 'dry fry' until the meat is sealed.
- Place all the other ingredients in the pan and simmer together for about 1–1½ hours.
- Serve with brown rice.

BEEF AND BEANS

SERVES 4

1 lb (450 g) lean stewing beef, cubed
1 medium onion, sliced
8 oz (225 g) carrots, diced
17 fl oz (500 ml) beef stock
dried or chopped fresh mixed herbs to taste
salt and freshly milled black pepper
1 × 14-oz (400-g) tin reduced-sugar baked beans

- Pre-heat the oven to gas mark 4, 350°F (180°C).
- Place the beef cubes and vegetables in a casserole dish. Add the stock, herbs and seasoning.
- Bake for 1 hour and then add the baked beans. Cook for further 30 minutes and serve.

STIR-FRY BEEF AND NOODLES

SERVES 1

4 oz (100 g) lean steak, with visible fat trimmed off
1 red pepper, de-seeded
½ onion
1 teaspoon soy sauce
1 teaspoon dry sherry or dry vermouth
1 teaspoon tomato purée
1 teaspoon wine vinegar
1 teaspoon sesame or sunflower oil
1 clove garlic, peeled and finely chopped
1 teaspoon peeled and finely chopped fresh root ginger
3 oz (75 g) Chinese noodles (preferably wholewheat)

✳ Cut the beef across the grain into very thin strips. Slice the red pepper and onion into bite-size pieces. Mix together the soy sauce, sherry or vermouth, tomato purée and wine vinegar.

✳ Heat the oil in a wok or heavy non-stick frying-pan. Add the onion, garlic and ginger and stir-fry for a minute; add the red pepper and continue to stir-fry for a further minute. Then add the beef and stir-fry for a further minute. Add 1 tablespoon water if things start to stick. (Don't cook any longer or the beef will toughen.)

✳ Add the soy sauce mixture, bring to the boil, stir well then serve immediately with the prepared noodles which take about 6 minutes to cook (follow the directions on the packet).

STIR-FRY BEEF AND BROCCOLI

This is a quick and easy 10-minute meal. Tastes good, too!

SERVES 1

4 oz (100 g) lean steak, fillet or rump or sirloin
4 oz (100 g) broccoli, fresh or frozen
½ small onion, roughly chopped
1 clove garlic, peeled and finely chopped
1 × 1-inch (2.5-cm) piece fresh root ginger, peeled and finely chopped
2 tablespoons oyster sauce or 1 tablespoon soy sauce and 1 tablespoon tomato ketchup (or tomato purée)
1 tablespoon dry sherry or dry vermouth or dry white wine or water
1–2 teaspoons wine or cider vinegar
¼ teaspoon Chinese five spice powder (optional)

❀ Slice the beef into thin strips across the grain. Break the broccoli into florets and cut the stems into bite-size pieces.

❀ 'Dry fry' (see p. 86) the onion, garlic and ginger for 1–2 minutes. Add 1 tablespoon water if it starts to stick.

❀ Add the beef and stir-fry for another minute.

❀ Add the broccoli and stir-fry for another 1–2 minutes.

❀ Mix all the other ingredients together and add to the pan. Stir well. Let it bubble for about 30 seconds and then serve.

STEAK WITH MUSTARD SAUCE

This is a very quick steak recipe. If you prefer more or less mustard then vary the amount used to taste.

SERVES 1

1 × 5-oz (150-g) sirloin, fillet or rump steak
2 tablespoons 8% fromage frais or Greek yoghurt (see p. 90)
½ teaspoon English mustard or 1 teaspoon Dijon or
Beaune mustard
salt and freshly milled black pepper

✤ Trim all visible fat from the meat.
✤ Heat a heavy non-stick frying-pan and 'dry fry' (see p. 86) the steak until it is done to your taste. Remove to a heated plate and keep warm.
✤ Add 1 tablespoon of water to the pan and scrape up any residue; then stir in the fromage frais (or yoghurt) and mustard and heat very gently. DO NOT BOIL. Season.
✤ Serve the steak with the sauce poured over.

CHUNKY VEGETABLES AND BEEF

SERVES 4

1 medium onion, chopped
12 oz (350 g) lean minced beef
7-oz (200-g) fresh or tinned tomatoes, chopped
10 fl oz (300 ml) beef stock
8 oz (225 g) shredded cabbage
8 oz (225 g) carrot, peeled and diced
1 small green or red pepper, de-seeded and chopped
salt and freshly milled black pepper

❋ Pre-heat the oven to gas mark 4, 350°F (180°C).
❋ 'Dry fry' (see p. 86) the onions until soft. Add the mince and seal it. Pour off any fat. Add all the other ingredients. Transfer to a casserole dish.
❋ Bake for 30 minutes.

CHILLI MINCE

SERVES 4

2 medium onions, finely chopped
1 lb (450 g) lean minced beef
¼–½ teaspoon hot chilli powder or to taste
2–3 teaspoons paprika
1 × 14-oz (400-g) tin red kidney beans, drained
1 lb (450 g) carrots, peeled and coarsely grated
1 × 14-oz (400-g) tin chopped tomatoes
salt and freshly milled black pepper

❋ 'Dry fry' (see p. 86) the onions until soft. Put in the minced beef and break it up well. Stir until the beef begins to brown.
❋ Add the chilli powder and paprika, lower the heat and continue cooking, stirring frequently, for 2 minutes. Pour off any fat.
❋ Mix in the red kidney beans and carrots. Add the tomatoes and bring to the boil. Add seasoning and stir well.
❋ Cover the saucepan and keep on a low heat for 30 minutes.

SHEPHERD'S PIE

SERVES 4

1 onion, chopped
1 lb (450 g) lean minced beef
10 fl oz (300 ml) beef stock
1 lb (450 g) potatoes
1 oz (50 g) cornflour
salt and freshly milled black pepper
2 fl oz (50 ml) skimmed milk
¾ oz (20 g) low-fat spread

❋ Pre-heat the oven to gas mark 6, 400°F (200°C).
❋ 'Dry fry' (see p. 86) the onions until soft. Add the meat and seal it. Pour off any fat. Add the stock, and cook over a low heat for 30 minutes, stirring from time to time.
❋ Meanwhile, peel the potatoes and boil them.
❋ Mix the cornflour with a tablespoon of cold water and then stir into the mince. Simmer until thickened. Season and pour into an ovenproof dish.
❋ Drain and mash the potatoes with the skimmed milk and low-fat spread. Spoon it onto the meat and 'fork' up the top. Bake for about 20 minutes or until golden brown.

BEEF CASSEROLE

SERVES 4

2 leeks, washed well and sliced
12 oz (350 g) swede
4 oz (100 g) pearl barley
1½ pints (900 ml) beef stock
4 carrots, peeled and sliced
1 lb (450 g) lean braising steak, trimmed of all fat and cut into strips
salt and freshly milled black pepper

❋ Pre-heat the oven to gas mark 3, 325°F (170°C).
❋ Put all the ingredients into a saucepan and bring to the boil. Skim the fat from the top of the pan. Stir well and put into a casserole.
❋ Cover and cook in the oven for 1–2 hours or until the meat is tender. Serve hot.

LAMB AND MINT KEBABS WITH YOGHURT SAUCE

As the minced lamb on sale tends to be quite fatty, for this dish use either neck fillet, lamb steak, or a lamb chop. Cut off the bone (if necessary) and trim off all visible fat.

SERVES 1
4 oz (100 g) lean lamb
1 clove garlic, peeled
2 tablespoons finely chopped fresh mint
salt and freshly milled black pepper
squeeze of lemon juice
2 tablespoons low-fat natural yoghurt

❋ Mince or process in a food processor the lamb, garlic and 1 tablespoon of the mint. Add salt, freshly milled black pepper and a squeeze of lemon juice.
❋ Using wet hands, shape the lamb into 3 or 4 small sausage shapes and thread onto a skewer.
❋ Grill the lamb fiercely for 6–8 minutes, turning twice.
❋ Mix the other tablespoon of mint into the yoghurt, season and serve with the lamb kebabs.

NOTE You can use left-over roast lamb for this – but again, trim it of every trace of fat.

LAMB'S KIDNEYS IN MUSHROOM SAUCE

This makes a quick, rich-tasting and satisfying dish. You can add 1 tablespoon of white wine or vermouth instead of the water – add it after you've fried the kidneys.

SERVES 1

4 oz (100 g) lamb's kidneys
½ small onion, finely chopped
1 clove garlic, peeled and finely chopped
2 oz (50 g) mushrooms, sliced
2 tablespoons 8% fromage frais or Greek yoghurt (see p. 90)
salt and freshly milled black pepper
squeeze of lemon juice (optional)
finely chopped fresh parsley to garnish

❋ Take the white core out of the kidneys and leave them in halves or cut them into quarters.

❋ 'Dry fry' (see p. 86) the onion and garlic until soft but not coloured, add the mushrooms and fry for a further 1–2 minutes until they are soft. Remove the onion and mushroom mixture from the pan.

❋ Add the kidneys to the pan and 'dry-fry' quickly for 1–2 minutes. It's best to leave them slightly pink inside – they are then more tender. Put the onion and mushrooms back into the pan, add 1 tablespoon of water to scrape up any residue, bring to the boil and then remove from the heat. Then add the fromage frais or Greek yoghurt and stir well. Heat gently but DO NOT BOIL.

❋ Season with salt, freshly milled black pepper and lemon juice, if you like, and serve sprinkled with parsley.

MARINATED LAMB CUTLETS
···

SERVES 1

6 oz (175 g) lamb cutlets (weight including bones)
juice of ½ lemon
2 tablespoons low-fat natural yoghurt
1 clove garlic, peeled and crushed
1 tablespoon finely chopped fresh oregano or fresh mint
or ½ teaspoon dried oregano or mint
salt and freshly milled black pepper
wedge of lemon

※ Trim all visible fat from the lamb.

※ Whisk together the lemon juice and yoghurt; stir in the garlic and herbs.

※ Place the trimmed cutlets in a shallow dish and pour the yoghurt marinade over them. Marinate for 6–24 hours, turning as often as you can.

※ Pre-heat a grill to its highest setting. Scrape the marinade off the cutlets. Grill quickly for 3–4 minutes, turning once. To keep them juicy, they should be browned on the outside but still pink inside.

※ Season and serve with a wedge of lemon.

LAMB PILAF
....

SERVES 1

2 oz (50 g) lamb, neck fillet or chump chop or 2 oz (50 g)
left-over cooked lamb
½ onion, finely chopped
2 oz (50 g) bulgar wheat (burghul, pourgouri, or cracked wheat)
2 oz (50 g) peas
2 teaspoons raisins or sultanas
salt and freshly milled black pepper
1 tablespoon low-fat natural yoghurt (optional)

✳ Remove all fat from the lamb and finely chop or mince the meat.

✳ 'Dry fry' (see p. 86) the onion until soft, add the bulgar wheat and stir and fry for a minute or so. If you are using raw lamb add it now and stir. Add a cup of water and the peas. Stir well. Simmer for 8–10 minutes until the wheat has swollen and is tender, adding more water if necessary.

✳ Towards the end of the cooking time, if you are using cooked lamb stir it in together with the raisins or sultanas. Heat thoroughly. When the bulgar wheat is cooked, season and serve, topped with the yoghurt if wished.

LAMB-STUFFED PEPPERS

SERVES 1

3 oz (75 g) lamb fillet or boneless chop or
3 oz (75 g) left-over lamb
½ onion, finely chopped
1–2 cloves garlic, peeled and finely chopped
2 oz (50 g) brown long-grain rice
2 oz (50 g) mushrooms, finely chopped
1 tablespoon chopped fresh dill (optional)
salt and freshly milled black pepper
squeeze of lemon juice
1 large red, yellow or green pepper, halved, de-cored
and de-seeded
1 tablespoon tomato purée
1–2 teaspoons wine or cider vinegar

✽ Trim the lamb of all fat and finely chop the meat. Pre-heat the oven to gas mark 4, 350°F (180°C).

✽ 'Dry fry' (see p. 86) the onion and garlic until soft. Stir in the brown rice and mushrooms and stir and fry for another minute or so. Stir in the lamb if you are using raw lamb. Add a cupful of hot water and start simmering.

✽ Simmer until the rice is cooked, adding more hot water – a half a cup at a time – as necessary. You should end up with the rice cooked and all the liquid evaporated except for a couple of tablespoons. If you are using cooked lamb, mix it in when the rice is cooked. Now stir in the dill, if you are using it. Season with salt, freshly milled black pepper and a squeeze of lemon juice.

✽ Place the pepper halves in an appropriate ovenproof dish and stuff them with the lamb and rice mixture. Mix the tomato purée and vinegar with 4 tablespoons of water and pour over and around the peppers.

✽ Bake in the oven for 25–30 minutes until the peppers are tender but not collapsed.

SALADS AND SALAD DRESSINGS

EACH SERVES 1

Here are some salad ideas. Where I haven't specified quantities, the amount you have is up to you – you can really eat your fill without worrying about the calories! I've suggested some salad dressings here, but of course you can use any of the salad dressings (pp. 325–8) with any of these salad ideas. I find that the simple combination of fresh lemon juice and fresh herbs is also a very good dressing.

TOMATO SALAD
❋ Sliced ripe tomatoes with Yoghurt, lemon and basil dressing (see p. 325).

ARAB SALAD
❋ A delicious refreshing mixture of cucumber, tomatoes and spring onions (see p. 245 for how to make it).

COLESLAW
❋ Grate or finely shred white cabbage, apple and carrot and add the Yoghurt, lemon and herb dressing (see p. 325) with parsley or chives. This keeps for a couple of days in the fridge and tastes much better than shop-bought coleslaw. If you do buy coleslaw, buy a lower calorie version.

MIXED LEAF SALAD
❋ A mixture of leaves like Cos, Little Gem, red oak leaf, frisée, radicchio or rocket tossed with Tomato vinaigrette (see p. 327).

BUTTON MUSHROOM SALAD
❋ White button mushrooms, wiped and very finely sliced and then mixed with Yoghurt, lemon and herb dressing (see p. 325).

SPICY TOMATO SALAD

❋ Sliced tomatoes and thinly sliced Spanish onions (previously soaked in cold water if you want them very mild) with Spicy tomato dressing (see p. 328).

'DIET WALDORF' SALAD

❋ Chunks of red apple, cucumber and celery, mixed with yoghurt and orange juice (1 tablespoon low-fat natural yoghurt to 1 teaspoon orange juice).

MINTY CUCUMBER SALAD

❋ Peeled or unpeeled cucumber grated or cut into chunks or slices and then mixed with the Yoghurt and mint dressing (see p. 326). This is a version of the Indian chutney called raita.

ROASTED PEPPER SALAD

❋ An unusual and tasty salad (see p. 239).

FENNEL AND RED PEPPER SALAD

❋ Slice the fennel and de-seed and cut the red pepper into strips. Dress with lemon juice or Tomato vinaigrette (see p. 327).

BEANSPROUTS AND PEPPER SALAD

❋ De-seed and thinly slice red, green or yellow pepper and mix with beansprouts. Serve with Chinese tomato dressing (see p. 328).

CARROT SALAD

❋ Grate or shred washed carrots and mix with Yoghurt, lemon and herb dressing (see p. 325): using dill or fennel is good, but any herb goes well.

CHINESE LEAF AND RADISH SALAD

✳ Shred the Chinese leaves (Chinese cabbage) thinly and cut the radishes into matchstick sized pieces. Serve with Spicy yoghurt dressing (see p. 325) or Spicy tomato dressing (see p. 328).

PEA SALAD

✳ Cook 3–4 oz (75–100 g) peas, drain and cool slightly. While they are still warm, mix with Yoghurt and mint dressing (see p. 326) and serve cold. You could add 1 or 2 finely chopped spring onions if you like.

BROAD BEAN SALAD

✳ Cook 3 oz (75 g) broad beans, drain and cool slightly. While they are still warm, mix with Yoghurt, lemon and herb dressing (see p. 325) or Spicy yoghurt dressing (see p. 325) and serve cold.

MANGETOUT SALAD

✳ Cook 3–4 oz (75–100 g) mangetout until they are cooked but still crisp. Drain, and cool slightly. Mix with Tomato vinaigrette (see p. 327) and serve cold.

In addition to the following dressings, see also low-calorie 'mayonnaise' or salad cream and its variations on p. 346. As well as using any of these for salads, you could also use them as toppings for baked potatoes.

If any of the yoghurt dressings are too thick for you, thin them down with a little skimmed milk. Instead of just yoghurt, you could also try using 1% fromage frais or even a combination of fromage frais and yoghurt.

YOGHURT, LEMON AND HERB DRESSING

1–2 tablespoons low-fat natural yoghurt
1–2 teaspoons lemon juice
½–1 tablespoon finely chopped fresh herbs such as parsley, chervil,
chives, tarragon, dill, fennel or basil
salt and freshly milled black pepper

✳ Whisk all the ingredients together. Season to taste.

NOTE Instead of lemon juice, you could use orange, apple or grapefruit juice or a smaller quantity of wine or cider vinegar.

SPICY YOGHURT DRESSING

½–1 teaspoon Dijon mustard
1 clove garlic, peeled and crushed or finely chopped
1–2 drops Tabasco sauce
1–2 tablespoons low-fat natural yoghurt
salt and freshly milled black pepper

✳ Whisk all the ingredients together. Season to taste.

SEAFOOD YOGHURT DRESSING

This pink sauce is good with any seafood, but particularly prawns.

1–2 teaspoons tomato ketchup or tomato purée
1 clove garlic, peeled and crushed or finely chopped
1–2 tablespoons low-fat natural yoghurt
1–2 drops Worcestershire sauce (optional)
1–2 teaspoons lemon juice
salt and freshly milled black pepper

✳ Whisk all the ingredients together. Season to taste.

YOGHURT TARTARE SAUCE

This is particularly good spread on a baked potato. It is also excellent served at the side of grilled, steamed or poached fish. As a salad dressing it's probably best thinned down with some skimmed milk.

2–3 spring onions, finely chopped
½ tablespoon finely chopped fresh parsley
½ dill cucumber or 2 gherkins, finely chopped
2 tablespoons low-fat natural yoghurt
lemon juice to taste
salt and freshly milled black pepper

✳ Mix all the ingredients together. Season to taste.

YOGHURT AND MINT DRESSING

This is also very good with a baked potato.

1–2 tablespoons low-fat natural yoghurt
½ tablespoon finely chopped fresh mint
½–1 clove garlic, peeled and crushed or finely chopped (optional)
salt and freshly milled black pepper
squeeze of lemon juice

✳ Mix everything together and season to taste with salt, pepper and lemon juice.

TOMATO VINAIGRETTE

This is a lovely dressing, thinner than a yoghurt dressing, and good with all salad things. Even plain lettuce is delicious with this. You can vary the fresh herbs used although basil is particularly good.

2 ripe tomatoes
1–2 teaspoons wine or cider vinegar or lemon juice
½ clove garlic, peeled and crushed or finely chopped (optional)
½–1 tablespoon finely chopped fresh basil (optional)
salt and freshly milled black pepper

✳ Skin the tomatoes by nicking at the core with a sharp knife, pouring over boiling water, leaving for 1 minute then plunging them into cold water. The skin can then be peeled off easily.

✳ Process the tomatoes and other ingredients in a liquidiser or food processor until smooth. Season to taste.

QUICK TOMATO DRESSING

1–2 tablespoons tomato juice or 1–2 teaspoons tomato purée
mixed with 3–6 teaspoons water
1–2 teaspoons lemon juice
salt and freshly milled black pepper

✳ Mix together the tomato and lemon juice and season.

SPICY TOMATO DRESSING

1–2 tablespoons tomato juice or *1–2 teaspoons tomato purée*
mixed with 3–6 teaspoons water
1 clove garlic, peeled and crushed or *finely chopped*
1–2 teaspoons lemon juice
Worcestershire sauce to taste
freshly milled black pepper

❋ Mix the ingredients together and season with Worcestershire sauce and freshly milled black pepper (salt probably won't be necessary).

CHINESE TOMATO DRESSING

1–2 tablespoons tomato juice or *1–2 teaspoons tomato purée*
mixed with 3–6 teaspoons water
1 clove garlic, peeled and sliced (optional)
1 × ½-inch (1-cm) piece fresh root ginger, peeled and sliced
(optional)
1–2 teaspoons soy sauce (or more to taste)
squeeze of lemon juice

❋ If you are using the garlic and ginger, leave them to soak in the tomato juice for as long as you can. Then drain, discarding the garlic and ginger.

❋ Mix together the tomato juice, soy sauce and lemon juice.

NOTE This is also good substituting orange juice for part of the tomato juice.

PUDDINGS

NOTE In the recipes where gelatine is used, don't be put off if you're uncertain about using it – it's really very easy.

THE BBC DIET CHOCOLATE MOUSSE

Chocolate mousse on a diet? Well this is a lighter than normal version but it's still very good and feels like a treat. Even though it's only half the calories of normal chocolate mousse, that's still quite a lot so, as you'll see from the diet plans, it's a once-a-week treat.

SERVES 4
4 oz (100 g) dark chocolate
2 eggs, separated (see p. 89)
6 oz (175 g) 1% fromage frais (see p. 90)

* Break the chocolate up into squares and place in a small bowl. Place the bowl in a small pan of water which has just boiled. Leave off the heat for 3 or 4 minutes until the chocolate has melted.
* Beat the egg yolks into the melted chocolate until smooth. Leave to cool slightly.
* Beat the egg whites until holding in peaks but not too stiff. Fold into the chocolate mixture. Then gently stir in the fromage frais.
* Pour into 4 small dishes or glasses and refrigerate until set.

APPLE CINNAMON TOAST

Cinnamon toast is of course a Victorian nursery favourite – but it's normally dripping with butter and sugar! Here's something inspired by it which makes a very quick and filling pudding.

SERVES 1
1 eating apple
1 slice wholemeal bread (about 1 oz/25 g)
¼ teaspoon or less of cinnamon
1 scant level teaspoon icing sugar

* Core and cut the apple into thin crescents.
* Toast one side of the bread and cut off the crusts.
* Cover the bread on the untoasted side with the apple slices and sprinkle with the sugar and cinnamon mixed together.
* Grill until it's browning.
* Serve with cold 1% fromage frais (see p. 90) or low-fat natural yoghurt if you like.

STRAWBERRY MOUSSE

This makes a solidly-set strawberry mousse. As an alternative, you could use raspberries instead of strawberries.

SERVES 4
6 oz (175 g) ripe strawberries
6 oz (175 g) low-fat natural yoghurt
6 oz (175 g) 1% fromage frais (see p. 90)
3 teaspoons powdered gelatine

* Liquidise together the strawberries, yoghurt and fromage frais.
* Sprinkle the gelatine into half a cup of very hot water. Stir briskly until it dissolves.

❋ Stir the gelatine into the strawberry mixture and pour into a wetted mould or bowl or into 4 individual serving dishes.

❋ Serve when set, topped, if you like, with more low-fat natural yoghurt.

ORANGES IN ORANGE JELLY

A happy variation of this is to use 8 oz (225 g) fresh strawberries in place of the citrus fruit.

SERVES 4

3 level teaspoons powdered gelatine
1 pint (600 ml) unsweetened orange juice
4 satsumas or tangerines or mandarins, peeled and segmented or
1 × 10-oz (275-g) tin mandarins, in natural juice, drained

❋ Sprinkle the gelatine into half a cup of very hot water. Stir briskly until it dissolves.

❋ Pour the gelatine mixture into the orange juice, mixing well as you pour.

❋ Let the mixture cool. Stir in whichever citrus fruit segments you are using and pour into a wetted mould or basin or 4 individual serving dishes.

❋ Serve when set, with low-fat natural yoghurt or 1% fromage frais (see p. 90) if you like.

APPLE JELLY WITH GRAPES
....

This is as easy to make as a packet of jelly.

SERVES 4

3 level teaspoons powdered gelatine
1 pint (600 ml) unsweetened apple juice
8 oz (225 g) grapes, seedless or *halved and de-seeded*

❋ Sprinkle the gelatine into half a cup of very hot water. Stir briskly until it dissolves.

❋ Pour the gelatine mixture into the apple juice, mixing well as you pour.

❋ Let the mixture cool, stir in the grapes and pour into a wetted mould or basin or 4 individual dishes.

❋ Serve when set, with some low-fat natural yoghurt or 1% fromage frais (see p. 90) if you like.

FRUIT KEBABS
....

SERVES 4

1 apple
1 pear
squeeze of lemon or *lime juice*
1 banana
2 satsumas or *tangerines* or *1 orange*
4 oz (100 g) grapes, seedless or *de-seeded*
2 teaspoons icing sugar

❋ Core the apple and pear and cut into bite-size pieces. Put in a bowl and sprinkle with the lemon or lime juice. Peel the banana and cut into 4. Peel and segment whichever citrus fruit you're using.

❋ Thread the pieces of fruit onto 4 or 8 wooden skewers, alternating the varieties.

❋ Sprinkle each skewer evenly with icing sugar. Place the skewers on a piece of kitchen foil if you like.

❋ Grill as quickly as possible under a grill pre-heated to its highest setting until the sugar just begins to caramelise and turn brown but the fruit is still firm.

❋ Serve hot with, if you like, low-fat natural yoghurt or 1% fromage frais (see p. 90).

NOTE Any other fruits could be used such as grapefruit, strawberries, peaches or mango.

SPICY PEAR AND ORANGE

SERVES 4

5 fl oz (150 ml) unsweetened orange juice

juice of 1 lemon

2 tablespoons water

¼ teaspoon ground ginger

¼ teaspoon cinnamon

1 lb (450 g) dessert pears, peeled, cored and sliced

❋ In a pan mix the juices with the water and spices, add the pears and bring to the boil and simmer gently until the pears are soft.

❋ Chill before serving.

CHOPPED APPLE CRUNCH

SERVES 1

1 slice wholemeal bread or 2 tablespoons rolled oats
5 oz (150 g) dessert apple, chopped (peeled if preferred)

❋ Toast the bread and make into breadcrumbs or grill the oats or toast them in the oven.
❋ Sprinkle the crumbs or oats over the apple. Serve alone or with low-fat natural yoghurt or 1% fromage frais (see p. 90).

BAKED APPLE WITH SULTANAS AND APPLE JUICE

Baked apples are much nicer using eating apples rather than so-called baking apples.

SERVES 1

1 large eating apple (Cox's are good)
½ oz (15 g) sultanas or raisins
5 tablespoons unsweetened apple juice or water
sprinkle of cinnamon (optional)

❋ Pre-heat the oven to gas mark 4, 350°F (180°C). Prepare a piece of foil which will comfortably envelop the apple.
❋ Core the apple and stuff with the sultanas or raisins. Place on the foil, pour over the apple juice and sprinkle with a little cinnamon if you like. Seal the foil tightly into a small parcel.
❋ Bake for about 15 minutes.
❋ Serve hot with cold low-fat natural yoghurt or 1% fromage frais (see p. 90) if you like.

NOTE You could also microwave this if you use greaseproof paper instead of foil. It takes about a minute on full power, but refer to your own microwave instruction book.

BAKED BANANA AND ORANGE

SERVES 1
1 banana
5 tablespoons unsweetened orange juice
grated nutmeg (optional)

✳ Pre-heat the oven to gas mark 4, 350°F (180°C). Prepare a piece of foil which will comfortably envelop the banana.
✳ Peel the banana and place on the foil. Pour over the orange juice and sprinkle with nutmeg if using. Seal the foil tightly into a small parcel.
✳ Bake for about 10 minutes.
✳ Serve hot with cold low-fat natural yoghurt or 1% fromage frais if you like (see p. 90).

NOTE You could also microwave this if you use greaseproof paper instead of foil. It takes about 45 seconds on full power, but refer to your own microwave instruction book.

PEAR AND TOFU WHIP

This has an interesting, grainy, almost nutty texture which makes a pleasant change from yoghurt textures! It is also quite filling. Use the solid block kind of tofu. (If you like, you could use 2 small bananas instead of the pears.)

SERVES 2
2 ripe but still firm pears
4 oz (100 g) firm tofu

✳ Core the pears but leave on the peel unless you hate it.
✳ Liquidise the tofu and pears together until you've got a thick smooth purée.
✳ Serve in small dishes or sundae glasses.

BANANA SPLIT

SERVES 1

1 banana
2 teaspoons 8% fromage frais (see p. 90)
2 teaspoons low-fat natural yoghurt
2 oz (50 g) ripe strawberries

* Peel the banana, cut into 2 lengthways and place in a suitable dish.
* Mix together the fromage frais and yoghurt and spoon between the 2 banana halves.
* Process or liquidise the strawberries or, alternatively, push them through a sieve. Pour the resulting strawberry sauce over the banana halves.

STRAWBERRIES WITH RASPBERRY SAUCE

This is based on a recipe by Delia Smith. Sorry Delia, I've left out the sugar and cream!

SERVES 2

8 oz (225 g) ripe strawberries
4 oz (100 g) ripe raspberries
4 teaspoons Greek yoghurt or 8% fromage frais (see p. 90)

* Hull the strawberries and arrange in 2 dishes.
* Process or liquidise the raspberries, or push them through a sieve. Pour the purée over the strawberries.
* Top each dish with 2 teaspoons of Greek yoghurt or fromage frais.

NOTE You could use larger quantities of low-fat natural yoghurt or 1% fromage frais.

GREEK FRUIT SALAD

*This is very simple, but it's somehow more interesting and satisfying
than taking your own fruit from a fruit bowl and peeling it. It makes
a spectacular and slimming end to a special meal.*

SERVES 4
*about a dozen ice cubes
selection of fruits (e.g. melon, watermelon, fresh figs, mango,
papaya (paw paw), grapes, strawberries, kiwi fruit), peeled and
sliced or left whole
juice of ½ lime or lemon*

❋ Crush the ice cubes in a food processor or put into a thick,
   plastic bag and bash with a rolling pin.
❋ Arrange the crushed ice on an attractive serving plate.
❋ Arrange the fruit and slices of fruit on top of the ice and
   sprinkle with the lime juice. Serve immediately.

DRIED FRUIT SALAD

SERVES 4
*8 oz (225 g) mixed dried fruit or use just one variety (e.g. apricots,
peaches, pears or prunes)
10 fl oz (300 ml) unsweetened apple juice*

❋ Place the fruit and apple juice in a small pan, bring slowly
   to the boil, simmer for 2 or 3 minutes and then leave to cool.
❋ If you like, serve with low-fat natural yoghurt or 1%
   fromage frais (see p. 90).

FRESH FRUIT SALAD

Fruit salad always seems more of a 'pudding' and more satisfying than fresh fruit eaten 'as it comes'. Serve this with low-fat natural yoghurt or 1% fromage frais (see p. 90).

SERVES 4
1 red apple
1 green apple
squeeze of lemon or lime juice
4 oz (100 g) black or green seedless grapes or stoned cherries
1–2 satsumas or tangerines or 1 orange
1 peach or nectarine or 2 apricots
5 fl oz (150 ml) unsweetened orange or apple juice

* Core the apples and, leaving the skin on, chop them into bite-size pieces. Squeeze a little lemon or lime juice on them.
* Add the grapes or cherries, the peeled and segmented satsumas, tangerines or orange, and the diced peach or nectarine or apricots.
* Pour the orange or apple juice over, stir well and try to leave for an hour or so to allow the flavours to merge before serving.

NOTE   Any fresh fruit can be used – pears, melon, strawberries or any you like. Bananas, I find, tend to go a bit soggy.

MANGO CREAM

Sorry – no actual cream, pace the Trades' Description Act! This makes a soft, unset, mousse-like pudding. The mango imparts a smooth unctuousness which makes it taste creamier than it is!

338

SERVES 4
1 ripe mango
8 oz (225 g) 1% fromage frais (see p. 90)
5 oz (150 g) low-fat natural yoghurt

❋ Cut the mango into 2 halves on either side of the large stone. Scrape out all the flesh (and juice!) into a liquidiser or food processor, scraping all the flesh too from the stone.
❋ Liquidise.
Put the processed mango into a bowl and stir in the fromage frais and low-fat natural yoghurt (this gives a better consistency than if you just liquidise everything together).
❋ Chill and serve, topped with more 1% fromage frais or low-fat natural yoghurt if you like.

APRICOT FOOL

If you wish you could also make Pineapple fool with 6–8 oz (175–225 g) fresh pineapple instead of the apricots or Passion fruit fool with the juice and pulp of 4 passion fruits and 4 teaspoons of caster sugar instead of the apricots.

SERVES 4
4 oz (100 g) dried apricots
8 oz (225 g) fromage frais
5 oz (150 g) low-fat natural yoghurt

❋ Put the apricots in a small saucepan and cover with water. Bring to the boil slowly and then simmer gently for 10–15 minutes. Leave to cool. The apricots should absorb most of the juice.
❋ Finely chop the apricots and their liquid in a liquidiser or food processor. Add the fromage frais and mix. Turn into a bowl and stir in the yoghurt until thoroughly blended.
❋ Serve in small bowls or glasses topped with a teaspoon of natural yoghurt.

SLIMMERS' LEMON CHEESECAKE
···

This has no (fattening!) base but has a lovely taste and texture. You can make it in individual dishes as it is difficult to cut and serve neatly. I'm grateful to Brynda Lewis, who assessed all the calorie counts of the diet plans, for this recipe.

SERVES 4
8 oz (225 g) cottage cheese
10 oz (275 g) low-fat natural yoghurt
1 oz (25 g) caster sugar
juice and finely grated rind of 1 small or ½ large lemon
3 teaspoons powdered gelatine

✱ Process or liquidise together the cottage cheese, yoghurt, sugar and lemon juice and rind.

✱ Dissolve the gelatine into half a cup of very hot water. Stir briskly.

✱ Mix the gelatine into the cottage cheese mixture, stirring well all the time.

✱ Pour into a wetted shallow dish or flan case or into individual dishes. Leave until set.

ORANGE OR APPLE BLANCMANGE

SERVES 4
5 oz (150 g) low-fat natural yoghurt
15 fl oz (450 ml) unsweetened orange or apple juice
3 level teaspoons powdered gelatine

❋ Put the yoghurt in a large bowl and whisk gently until smooth; pour in the orange or apple juice and mix thoroughly.

❋ Sprinkle the gelatine into half a cup of very hot water. Stir briskly.

❋ Pour the gelatine mixture into the yoghurt and fruit juice, stirring well as you pour.

❋ Pour into a wetted mould or bowl or into 4 individual serving dishes.

❋ Serve when set.

SIDE DISHES, SAUCES AND STOCK

POTATO GRATIN

This is a very quick version of the famous 'gratin dauphinois' and contains a fraction of the calories. For the quantity of potatoes you should have, see the instructions in the diet plan you are following.

SERVES 1

5–9 oz (150–250 g) potatoes, preferably waxy yellow ones
1–1½ tablespoons 8% fromage frais (see p. 90)
1–1½ tablespoons skimmed milk
½–1 clove garlic, peeled and finely chopped
salt and freshly milled black pepper

* Pre-heat the oven to gas mark 4, 350°F (180°C).
* Peel the potatoes and slice them thinly into rounds – each about the thickness of a two-pence coin.
* Mix together the fromage frais and milk, stir in the garlic and season.
* Add the potato slices and mix well so that each slice is coated.
* With a piece of kitchen paper dipped in oil, lightly grease a small ovenproof dish. Neatly layer the potatoes in the dish.
* Bake in the oven for 40–50 minutes or until the potatoes are cooked and the top is browned.

POTATOES BAKED WITH LEMON AND GARLIC

As for the Potato gratin, you need to check the quantity of potatoes you can eat by looking at the instructions in your chosen diet plan.

SERVES 1

5–9 oz (150–250 g) potatoes, preferably waxy yellow ones
½–1 clove garlic, peeled and finely chopped
juice and finely grated zest of up to ½ lemon
salt and freshly milled black pepper
2½–5 fl oz (65–150 ml) Chicken stock (see p. 348) or vegetable stock
finely chopped fresh parsley to garnish (optional)

✳ Pre-heat the oven to gas mark 4, 350°F (180°C).
✳ Peel the potatoes and slice them thinly into rounds – each about the thickness of a two-pence coin.
✳ Layer the potatoes in a small ovenproof dish, scattering a little garlic, lemon zest and salt and freshly milled black pepper on each layer.
✳ Mix together the stock and lemon juice and pour over the potatoes. (The potatoes should be just covered.)
✳ Bake in the oven for about 40–50 minutes or until the potatoes are soft and the top is browning.
✳ Serve, scattered with a little chopped parsley if you like.

NOTE As a variation, you could interleave a finely sliced onion with the potatoes.

RATATOUILLE

This does contain a tablespoonful of oil but, as it's shared among four people, it's not adding to the calorie count significantly.

SERVES 4

1 tablespoon olive or sunflower oil
2 medium courgettes, cut into ¼-in (5-mm) slices
3 medium tomatoes, quartered or 1 × 7-oz (200-g) tin tomatoes
1 medium aubergine, cut into 1-inch (2.5-cm) pieces
1 clove garlic, peeled and crushed
1 small onion, sliced
1 teaspoon dried mixed herbs or 1 tablespoon chopped mixed fresh herbs
salt and freshly milled black pepper

* Heat the oil in a large saucepan.
* Add half the vegetables and sauté for 1–2 minutes.
* Add the remaining vegetables and sauté for a further minute. Then simmer for 15 minutes, stirring occasionally.
* Add the herbs and seasoning. Simmer for 20 minutes, stirring occasionally, until the vegetables are soft.

FRESH TOMATO AND ONION CHUTNEY

SERVES 1

1 large or 2 small tomatoes
2 teaspoons finely chopped onion or spring onions
juice of ½ lemon or lime
salt and freshly milled black pepper
1 teaspoon paprika (optional)
¼ teaspoon chilli powder (optional)

* Finely chop the tomato and mix well with all the other ingredients. Try to leave for at least 30 minutes before serving to allow the flavours to merge.

BASIC LOW-CALORIE WHITE SAUCE
(BECHAMEL SAUCE)

This is an extremely easy sauce to make (as easy as any packet sauce). It tastes good and, as you can see, lends itself to several variations.

SERVES 1
5 fl oz (150 ml) cold skimmed milk
½ oz (15 g) low-fat spread (such as Gold or Outline)
½ oz (15 g) plain flour
salt and freshly milled black pepper

❋ Place the milk, then the low-fat spread and flour into a small saucepan (weigh out the low-fat spread and flour carefully).

❋ Place the pan over a moderate heat and heat the sauce whisking ALL THE TIME with a balloon or spiral coil whisk. (You may need to alternate with an angled wooden spoon to ensure you reach the corners of the pan.)

❋ When the sauce comes to the boil, turn the heat down to its lowest setting and simmer very gently for 2–3 minutes, stirring 4 or 5 times.

❋ Season with salt and freshly milled black pepper. If the texture is a little too thick for your taste, whisk in 1 or 2 tablespoons of skimmed milk.

PARSLEY SAUCE

❋ At the end of the cooking time stir in 2 tablespoons of finely chopped fresh parsley and 1 or 2 teaspoons of lemon juice.

MUSTARD SAUCE
This is delicious with fish or grilled chicken.

❋ Stir in at the end ½ teaspoon of English or (better, I think) 1 teaspoon of Dijon mustard.

CHEESE SAUCE
* Stir in at the end ½ teaspoon of Dijon or French mustard and 1 oz (25 g) finely grated low-fat (14%) Cheddar.

MUSHROOM SAUCE
* 'Dry fry' (see p. 86) 2 oz (50 g) chopped mushrooms with, if you like, 1 finely chopped peeled clove of garlic until they are soft and their juices are running. Stir into the sauce with 1–2 teaspoons of lemon juice.

ONION SAUCE
* 'Dry fry' (see p. 86) ½ finely chopped onion until soft, adding a tablespoon of water as you need to. Stir the onion into the sauce.

LOW-CALORIE 'MAYONNAISE' OR SALAD CREAM

This sounds rather unusual, but have faith: it's surprisingly good, especially if you use one of the flavour variations suggested. It's richer than, and therefore a pleasant change from, yoghurt dressings. It keeps for a couple of days in the fridge.

SERVES 2
1 quantity of White sauce made with 5 fl oz (150 ml) skimmed milk (p. 345)
3 tablespoons low-fat natural yoghurt
1 teaspoon wine or cider vinegar or lemon juice
½ teaspoon Dijon mustard (optional)
salt and freshly milled black pepper

* Make up the White sauce and leave to cool slightly.
* Then whisk in the yoghurt, vinegar (or lemon juice) and

mustard, if using. (You may prefer to add more or less vinegar or lemon juice according to taste.) Taste and season.
* Refrigerate for 1–2 hours before using.

GARLIC SAUCE
* Mix in with the yoghurt 1 or 2 finely crushed peeled cloves of garlic.

HERB SAUCE
* Mix in with the yoghurt 2 tablespoons of finely chopped herbs. Choose one herb – like parsley, tarragon, chives, basil or chervil – or a mixture.

'MARIE-ROSE' SAUCE (prawn cocktail sauce)
This is actually much better than many of the bottled sauces which masquerade under this name. It's good with crab, prawns or cold fish.
* Whisk in with the yoghurt 1 tablespoon of tomato ketchup or tomato purée.

CHICKEN STOCK
....

Any of the recipes in this book can be made with chicken stock from a cube if you prefer (though I don't think that something like Avgolemono on p. 234 would taste so good). Chicken stock is really so easy to make, tastes so much better, and is so convenient to have at hand if you freeze it in the way I suggest, that I really would encourage you to make it. After all, the idea is to have food with the least possible calories, not the least possible taste!

Those of us who don't run professional kitchens can happily make chicken stock out of chicken carcasses rather than whole chickens, but if you do poach a chicken (a very good way of cooking one), you'll get as a bonus a good stock. By the way, don't tell anyone who may come for a meal chez moi, but I always save gnawed chicken bones to put into my stock – they're as sterile as Dettol after this amount of boiling! You can save up the chicken carcasses in plastic bags in the freezer, and make up the stock when you've got 2 or 3 carcasses.

1 (or more) chicken carcasses and associated bones
½ onion (optional)
few sprigs of parsley (optional)
sprig of thyme (optional)
½ stick celery (optional)
bay leaf (optional)

* Simply break the carcass up, add any flavourings (it works fine without any) and cover with cold water.
* Bring to the boil and then simmer for about an hour.
* Strain the stock (discarding – finally – the carcass etc.) into a clean pan and boil hard until it has reduced by over half.
* Pour into a basin or bowl and refrigerate overnight. You should get a set jelly topped with a layer of fat. You know, of course, what you're going to do about the fat? That's right, scrape it all off. Every bit of it – then your stock is really low-calorie.

❋ Now boil up the stock and reduce by half again (watch it at the end). Now you should be left with about ½ a cup per chicken carcass of rich savoury stock. Pour this into a small bowl or cup and refrigerate until set.

❋ Now cut the set stock up into cubes of jelly. Cut the stock from one carcass into 4–6 cubes. Each of these when you come to use it should be dissolved in about 5 fl oz (150 ml) of water.

❋ Freeze the cubes, place in plastic bags and label.

20 Eating Out and Entertaining

OUT AND ABOUT

There are two ways of approaching a meal out when you're on *The BBC Diet*: controlling yourself or letting yourself go.

If you've gone out for a special occasion, I see no problem in having anything you want to eat. Why not enjoy yourself to the full? You can be 'off' your diet for one night and then back on it again the next day.

On the other hand, if you have to eat out often, you can't afford to take this liberal attitude – meals out two or three times a week can wreak havoc with your diet. Or you may feel that the fleeting enjoyment of a meal isn't worth delaying the day you reach your ideal weight.

If you're going out to a friend's house, it's sensible to say when you're accepting the invitation that you don't want to eat too much fattening food. This may be a challenge to a friend who's a keen cook to come up with something pleasing and low in calories – maybe you could send an advance present copy of *The BBC Diet*! If you are faced with food you'd rather not eat too much of, do remember how discouraging it is if you've been slaving over cooking to have someone refuse food. Your tactic in this situation should not be to refuse, but to ask for a small helping. If you really get a small helping, you can eat it all; if you don't, you can leave some. Obviously, don't add things like butter to your bread or cream to your pudding. Above all, remember that you can make up for a few hundred calories too many over the following week. I can't emphasise enough that it's what we eat *most* of the time that makes us fat, not what we eat occasionally.

If you're going to eat in a restaurant then you're more in control. Before you go, it's a good idea to read through the guidelines so they're fixed in your mind. Here are some other thoughts that can flash through it as you read the menu:

* Steer clear of alcohol. Apart from the calories it also encourages you to eat more. Remember how chic a mineral water with ice and lemon is.

* Don't eat the nibbles with the drinks.

* You should be able to spot a low-calorie first course – melon, grapefruit, clear soup are all perfect choices. As you look at each item ask yourself, 'Does this contain fat?' (perhaps even 'Does this contain sugar?'!) Remember avocado is quite high in calories and usually comes with an oily dressing. Hummus and taramasalata are usually full of oil. If there is something 'salady' make sure you ask if you can have it without the dressing.

* Ask for wholemeal bread; don't be tempted to put butter on it.

* For your main course you should, on the whole, look for something as simple as possible. The general rule is – the more human ingenuity has been at work on it, the more calories it contains (unless your chef follows Anton Mosimann's principles of *cuisine naturelle, naturellement*).

  Choose grilled fish, grilled chicken or a small grilled steak. Cut off the chicken skin and any visible fat on the steak. Say that you want it absolutely plain (ask for a slice of lemon to flavour it); make sure *maître d'* or any other kind of butter goes nowhere near it.

* Ask for a baked potato, or new potatoes, without added butter. You could try asking for low-fat yoghurt or low-fat spread for your baked potato. Boiled rice is a possibility. Make sure that your vegetables come neat – ask beforehand as often they come swimming in fat. If you're having a salad, again stress that you don't want any dressing. Trust your lemon slice again.

* For dessert, your best bet is fresh fruit. All restaurants should be able to provide this. Fresh fruit salad (no cream) would be an alternative but it's often quite sugary. Sorbet would be another reasonable bet. Avoid cheese – you'd probably eat too much. Of course, you're not even going to look at a sweet trolley.

* Don't put cream in your coffee. Often this is all that is offered. Ask for skimmed milk – you should get ordinary milk at least.

* Don't start nibbling the mints or chocolates they bring with the coffee.

* If you're having an Indian or Chinese meal, you should do well as the eating is usually communal. Make sure you have plain boiled rice and just taste small helpings of the other dishes.

AT HOME

Entertaining at home is easier than eating out because you're in complete control. It is possible to give your guests healthy, slimming food without their knowing it. If you entertain the same people regularly, you should certainly be concerned that what you're giving them is reasonably healthy. It's also helping you to stick to your diet while tucking in with abandon. Either follow recipes which you know are low in calories (like the ones in this book) or adapt them so that they conform to The BBC Diet guidelines.

If, on the other hand, you want to give your guests a real blow-out, make sure you leave somewhere in the meal for you to retreat to!

* Serve carrot, pepper and celery sticks as alternative nibbles with drinks.

* Serve sauces and dressings separately so you don't need to have them. The same goes for butter and cream.

* Always serve fresh fruit as well as puddings so you (or others) can say, 'I'm full but can manage a few grapes'. Fresh fruit salad in unsweetened fruit juice is the alternative.

Adapting Recipes

If you keep 'thinking fat and thinking sugar' you should be able to adapt many of your favourite recipes so that they contain far fewer calories.

* Gradually cut down the amount of sugar you add in recipes and aim to get down to half your normal quantity of sugar.

* Cutting the fat and the sugar in half works in most baking recipes.

* Substitute skimmed milk for whole milk and fromage frais or low-fat natural yoghurt for cream. (If you're heating yoghurt remember that a teaspoon of cornflower mixed with milk and stirred in should ensure that it doesn't curdle.)

* In all chicken recipes remove the skin.

* Always choose lean meat and trim off the fat.

* With soups, stocks and casseroles always try to prepare in advance. If you leave them to cool, the fat rises to the top and can be spooned off.

* After frying, pour off any fat and perhaps blot it up also with kitchen paper.

* But, preferably, of course you won't be frying! Think – can I grill? If not, 'dry-fry' (see p. 86) in a heavy non-stick frying-pan. If that's not possible, stir-fry in minimal oil and blot up the excess later.

* Whenever there's fat in a recipe ('1 oz, 25 g, butter', '4 tablespoons oil'), always halve it, at least. Better still, try it without.

21 Exercise and Speed Up Your Weight Loss!

If we compare ourselves to our recent ancestors, we are far less physically active than they were. It's not that we eat more than they did but we have cars, electric lawnmowers, automatic washing machines, vacuum cleaners, remote control televisions and, however useful they are, they are designed to stop us burning up calories! 'Convenience' equals not using our muscles as much as we would otherwise. Now this might seem insignificant, but added together and over months and years, the effects of our automated lifestyle do begin to count. A few dozen calories not burnt up in a day become a few pounds put on over the months, and stones over the years.

Our bodies were designed to be physically active on a regular basis. Without regular exercise they start to resemble badly tuned engines. You don't need to become a super-athlete, but your daily activity should be enough to get your body tuned up.

Later in this chapter are some suggestions for increasing the amount of your physical activity during the day. No matter how busy you are, you should be able to fit in some of them. Then, if you can – and you should certainly try – start to set some time aside for exercise. If you're overweight, the very best exercises you could begin with are walking or swimming and there are suggestions on these later, too. Also, there are some simple stretching and bending exercises which are going to help tone and firm up specific groups of muscles – in particular, your tummy, your buttocks, your bust, your thighs and your hips.

HOW BEING MORE ACTIVE HELPS YOU LOSE WEIGHT

Exercise does in itself burn up calories. Any physical activity burns up calories. When you're lying in bed, your body is ticking over at its basal metabolic rate or BMR (see p. 40). As soon as you start moving – walking downstairs, brushing your teeth, doing the ironing – you start burning up extra calories.

You may have heard that you have to take a lot of exercise to burn up a significant number of calories. But I'm not suggesting you try to burn off thousands in a day! A small daily increase in the number of calories you use up can have significant effects over a period of time. For example, if you carried on eating the way you were doing now and just started walking an extra mile a day, you could lose a pound a month, nearly a stone a year. So, that's the power of exercise without any dieting!

If you took it slowly, that mile might take you 20 minutes to walk. Instead of one 20-minute walk, you could use up the same number of calories doing 20 one-minute walks or 40 30-second walks. That is why it's important to look through the suggestions on p. 360 and try to think how you can build more mini- or micro-walks into your daily life.

As well as the burning-up of the calories as you actually exercise, there's evidence that regular, sustained exercise can increase the tickover, the BMR, of your body. That means your body becomes more efficient at getting rid of those calories when you are resting – even when you are sleeping! The effect may not be very large, but it could be significant and certainly may help to counter that unfortunate tendency of your BMR to go down when you start dieting (see p. 40).

As well as this increase in the BMR, regular, sustained exercise may help improve the ability of the body to carry out thermogenesis, or burning up excess calories as heat (see p. 40).

So, as you can see, exercising as well as dieting gives you a further three-pronged attack on those excess pounds!

OTHER BENEFITS OF EXERCISE FOR DIETERS

* Exercise helps to tone up all the muscles of your body. Even before you've lost all the weight you want to, this increased muscle tone helps to improve the shape of your body.

* Regular exercise helps to increase the amount of lean muscle in your body at the expense of the fat tissue.

* People who don't exercise think that exercise tends to increase the appetite. It doesn't. Most people who exercise regularly find that exercise tends to depress the appetite for an hour or so afterwards. I certainly find this is true. So think of the advantage of exercise before meal-times!

* Exercise becomes an enjoyable activity. It's also something to do other than eating. Going for a walk is a good diversion tactic if you're tempted by some fatty or sugary food.

OTHER HEALTH BENEFITS OF EXERCISE

* With an increase in physical activity, you'll start to feel better in yourself. Most people find they feel at their peak when they exercise regularly. It doesn't take much exercise to help you feel 'tuned-up'.

* Exercise is a great – and natural – way of relieving stress.

* Increasing your physical activity will help you to sleep more soundly.

* Regular use helps your joints and muscles to remain supple and keeps them working right into old age.

* Exercise helps to strengthen the bones and helps to delay or prevent osteoporosis, or thinning of the bones.

* Regular exercise helps to keep your blood pressure normal or helps to reduce it if it is too high.

* Regular exercise helps to strengthen your heart and enables it to have a bigger reserve capacity.

* Regular exercise helps to reduce the level of fats including cholesterol in your blood and so helps to cut the risk of heart attacks and strokes.

HOW CAN YOU RESIST ALL THESE BENEFITS?

Anyone can think of several excuses not to exercise, but compared with the benefits, they're all pretty flimsy.

* *I really am far too fat.* Being overweight really is an excellent reason and incentive to start exercising – it's going to help you to achieve your ideal weight.

* *I'm too tired.* Regular exercise will help you feel less tired! You'll find you'll have a lot more energy and, sleeping better, will wake up refreshed.

* *I'm too old.* You're never too old to exercise. Of course, as you get older you can't exercise as vigorously, but as long as you're puffing a little, you're getting the maximum benefit. Regular exercise also helps to ensure a more active old age.

* *I feel fine.* How you feel is a good indication of your health, but it's not the whole story: exercise will help you

to be healthy. And no matter how well you feel, you'll feel better when you exercise regularly.

✱ *I'm too busy.* If you're not used to putting aside time to exercise, you may find it difficult to fit into a busy life but see p. 360 for suggestions. Assess your priorities: isn't losing weight important to you? Don't think of exercise as a chore and it will become a pleasure, helping you to relax and cope more easily with work pressures and a busy life.

✱ *I'm not sporty.* You don't need to be as there are exercises to suit everyone. Walking and swimming are two of the very best. If you do want to take up a particular sport remember that exercise doesn't need to be competitive or championship-level to give the maximum benefit.

✱ *I've heard exercise is dangerous.* Of course, some people will have a heart attack while jogging; but far more will have one lying in bed or sitting watching television! If a middle-aged person, whose arteries are already partially clogged, suddenly starts taking vigorous exercise, he or she runs an increased risk of a heart attack. But, built up gradually, exercise is not only safe it will also help to protect you against a heart attack and improve your health in so many other ways. Someone who dies jogging might have died even earlier if he hadn't exercised at all!

✱ *I've got medical problems.* Obviously, if you're unfit and haven't exercised for a long time, you'd be wise to take it slowly and gently at first. You should consult your doctor first if you've suffered, or are suffering, from any of the following or are worried about any other aspect of your health:

high blood pressure or heart disease
chest problems like asthma or bronchitis
back trouble or a slipped disc
joint pains or arthritis
recuperation from illness or an operation

In all these conditions, the right exercise will help you to be healthier, but it's wise to ask your doctor's advice. If you've got a cold, 'flu, a sore throat or a temperature, it's wise not to exercise until you feel better.

Most people, even older people, don't need a medical check-up before starting regular exercise. Indeed, some American doctors would say you need a check-up if you *don't* exercise!

GETTING INTO A ROUTINE OF MORE ACTIVITY

What about beginning to think of some ways you could start to build more physical activity into your everyday life? Over a period of time, remember that quite small things can have a noticeable effect (see p. 356). First, keep an activity record for yourself for a couple of days. Look at the example on p. 361 (and see pages 407 and 408 for blank versions). You may be surprised by how little activity you undertake in a day.

After you've looked at your activity record, resolve on six or so things you're going to do immediately to start increasing the amount of physical activity you undertake in a day. Write them down (there is a blank version of an exercise diary on pages 409 and 410). The list below should give you some ideas. Each day, consider how well you've done.

* Walk to the station or walk part of the way.

* Get off the bus one or two stops earlier and walk the rest of the way.

* Cycle to work or to the shops or just for pleasure.

EXERCISE DIARY

	Where was I?	What did I do?
7.00	In bed	Switched alarm off
7.30	In bathroom	Showered, brushed teeth
8.00	In bedroom	Dressed; turned over pages of the newspaper
8.30	In kitchen	Ate breakfast
9.00	In car	Walked 3 yards to car and 10 yards from car to office
9.30	In office sitting at desk	Telephoned, wrote, walked 20 yards to the loo
10.00		
10.30		
11.00		
11.30		
12.00		
12.30	Eating sandwiches	Moving hands to mouth!
1.00		
1.30		
2.00	In office sitting at desk	Telephoning, writing, walked 5 yards to another office twice
2.30		
3.00		
3.30		
4.00		
4.30		
5.30	In car	Walked 10 yards from office to car; 3 yards from car to front door
6.00	In garden	Sitting
6.30		
7.00	In kitchen	Eating and drinking – moving hands to mouth!
7.30		
8.00	In the sitting room	Watching TV – pressing remote control switch!
8.30		
9.00		
9.30		
10.00	In bed	Reading – turning pages
10.30		
11.00	In bed	Asleep – tossing and turning!

* Walk to the shops; if you have a lot of shopping to carry, you could get someone to come to give you a lift back or take the bus back.

* Before you go for a bus or get the car out, think 'can I walk instead?'

* Use stairs instead of lifts or escalators whenever you can, remembering that although going up is tougher, you're burning more calories that way.

* Do some gardening or some more gardening. Mow the lawn more often.

* Walk the dog morning, noon and night if you can.

* At work, walk to someone else's office if you need to speak to them; don't use the phone.

* Keep thinking to yourself 'the more I move, the more calories I'll burn up and the sooner I'll get to my ideal weight'.

WALKING

For most people, walking is one of the very best ways of exercising: you don't need any special equipment, you don't need to be an expert, you don't need any coaching, you don't need to pay any money and you don't have to book time in a leisure centre. You can do it anytime, anywhere. Even if you're unfit and it's a long time since you've exercised, gentle walking can be your ideal way to increase your physical activity, to get fitter, and to burn up more calories.

In spite of the proclaimed virtues of jogging and other more 'sporty' activities, walking can get you just as fit and make you feel as good as any more vigorous sport – provided you walk for long enough and that you keep at it.

If it's a long time since you did any exercise, start by

walking for 5 or 10 minutes once or twice a day. Don't worry if you get a little bit out of puff. In fact, after a week or so, start walking a little faster so you get out of puff a little more. Getting a little out of breath is a good sign and means you're getting the maximum benefit. If you're very unfit, even a 5-minute walk could get you a little breathless, but you'll find, as you get fitter, you'll have to walk further, faster and perhaps even uphill a little before you start getting out of breath. This is good and is the sign that you're getting fitter.

Make sure you don't get so out of breath that you begin to feel uncomfortable; you should still be able to carry on a conversation if you wanted to. Stop if you feel uncomfortable or in any pain.

What you should aim to do is increase the length of time you walk by 5 minutes a day so that after a few weeks you're up to 20 minutes, 25 minutes then 30 minutes of brisk walking in each session. A 30- or 35-minute brisk walking session at least three times a week is ideal; if you're getting a little out of puff, you're doing as much as you need to do to get the maximum benefit for your health.

SWIMMING

In some ways swimming is an even better exercise than walking for people who are overweight. Because your body weight is supported by the water, there's no strain on your joints. The snag with swimming, of course, is that it takes a little more organisation than walking, but it is so enjoyable. Swimming is great for people of all ages and is good even if your back aches or you have joint pains. And it's something you can do with the whole family.

Some people who are overweight are embarrassed to go swimming – though there's a very wide array of body shapes and sizes on display at my local pool! If you feel shy, why not go in the early morning when few people are around?

Or, see if your local swimming baths have sessions for middle-aged or older people, or for women only, so you're not bothered by boisterous youngsters. If you've got a few friends who want to lose weight or go swimming together, why not think of hiring the swimming pool for half an hour or so? This is not as extravagant as you might think. In quiet times (like outside school holidays) you might find your local pool only too willing to let you do this. Often the cost is extremely reasonable.

Your aim in swimming is the same as for walking: to work up to a sustained 30-minute session in which you're comfortably a bit out of puff. Again, if you're unfit you should work up to this gradually over a period of a few weeks, adding 5 minutes extra each week.

WHAT ELSE CAN YOU DO?

I've mentioned walking and swimming in more detail because I think that they really are the best forms of exercise for people who are overweight. However, as you start losing weight and getting fitter, the world is your oyster and I really would advise you to start trying out some other sports or exercises that you feel you would enjoy.

Running or jogging

A jog is really just a slow run. Again, you need to go slowly for several weeks, at first alternating jogging with walking (see the chart on pp. 368–9). Build up gradually so that you're doing more jogging than walking and then all jogging. Don't get too breathless. You're not in a race, so don't increase your speed until you're ready. The time you spend jogging is more important in burning up calories than the speed at which you jog.

Try to run on grass as it's easier on your feet. You do need to buy a good pair of running shoes: go to a specialist sports shop and ask for advice. You'll get a lot of advice and help too if you join an athletics club. Jogging with a friend of approximately the same standard will encourage you to do it on a regular basis and not to skip it if you don't feel like it on a particular day.

Cycling

Again this may be a pleasant pastime for the whole family, or you could start cycling to work. Cycling is good exercise for those who are overweight, as their body weight is supported. To ensure you get sufficient exercise, get your legs moving hard and rhythmically. Build up gradually and increase the length of time you cycle by 5 minutes each week. Make sure you know your Highway Code and at night wear reflective clothing.

Badminton, tennis and squash

Badminton and tennis can be fun to play even if you're a beginner and again the whole family can join in. You get maximum benefit, though, as your play improves and you're playing against people of a similar or higher standard. Then the exercise will become more aerobic with fewer stops and starts. Singles tennis is likely to be more vigorous than doubles.

You should already be fit when you start playing squash; it can be a fast, hard game, but it is very efficient at burning off calories. If you're over 35, get fit with some other exercise before you start playing squash, and then begin by playing very gently.

Dancing

Waltzing isn't going to burn off too many calories though vigorous disco dancing will. Aerobic dancing classes, however, do provide a way of getting exercise which is of benefit to the heart. Some of them have been criticised for pushing people too quickly and so causing injuries or sprains, but some people enjoy exercising in company and find it encourages them to keep going. If you begin gradually, it's a good way of getting exercise. But do make sure your teacher is qualified.

Keep-fit classes and work-outs

If you want to do work-outs – bending and stretching exercises – you'll find that by far the best way of keeping at it is by going to keep-fit classes. It can get rather boring on your own. Some keep-fit classes are run especially for people who are overweight. Others, like step classes, are very vigorous. You may find you need to have already lost some weight, and to be reasonably fit, before you join one.

Make sure that you're getting reasonably breathless though – gently waving your arms around doesn't count as aerobic exercise! With this sort of keep-fit group, you burn off more calories walking briskly there and back home!

To get the most benefit, your exercise needs to be regular and sustained. Of course, you can vary the exercise: one day playing tennis, one day walking, one day swimming. If all this sounds too energetic for you, remember that anything is better than nothing. If only 1 or 2 sessions of exercise is possible, start there but do try to build up from it. For a detailed exercise plan see pp. 368–9.

GETTING INTO SHAPE AT HOME

If you don't want to exercise in public, you can burn off those calories in the privacy of your own home. Most of these solitary activities are rather boring and repetitive but you can always listen to music or the radio at the same time, have a conversation, or even watch television.

* skipping with a rope is superb aerobic exercise. Ten minutes quick skipping burns up 100 calories! However, it is very strenuous and you should start gently.

* running on the spot will also provide good exercise but is rather more boring.

* repeatedly going up and down stairs is good aerobic exercise – but you need to check your pulse rate with this as it's an exercise which will rapidly increase your heart rate.

* stationary bikes and rowing machines will give you excellent exercise. The very cheap ones are rather flimsy, so spend a bit more money – that will encourage you to use the thing as well! The best kinds of exercise bikes have adjustable pedal resistance so that you can work harder as you get fitter. Be sure you're really going to use one before you buy.

Apart from being private, all these activities are useful if you have a busy life and can't see where exercise would fit in.

In addition, here are some suggested exercises for suppleness which are also good for warming up before you do any more strenuous exercise and also exercises to help firm up some particular muscle groups (tummy, hips and thighs).

SUGGESTIONS FOR AN EXERCISE PLAN

Try do one session five days a week. The figures given
indicate minutes per session.

		Week 1	Week 2
Brisk Walking	Unfit	5	10
	Fit	10	20
Swimming	Unfit	5	10
	Fit	10	15
Skipping	Unfit	3	4
	Fit	2 x 5	10
Rowing & Cycling Machine	Unfit	5	7
	Fit	10	12
Aerobics Dancing	Unfit	5	8
	Fit	20	25
Cycling	Unfit	5	7
	Fit	15	20
Jogging	Unfit	Don't jog – 5 brisk walking	5 Alternate 15 secs jogging & 15 secs brisk walking
	Fit	10 Alternate 10 secs jogging & 10 secs brisk walking	15 Alternate 30 secs jogging & 30 secs brisk walking

Week 3	Week 4	Week 5	Week 6
15	20	25	30
25	25	30	35
15	20	25	30
20	25	30	35
5	6	7	8
2 x 6	15	2 x 9	20
10	12	15	20
15	20	25	30
10	12	15	20
30	40	50	60
10	15	20	25
25	30	35	40
10 Alternate 30 secs jogging & 30 secs brisk walking	15 Alternate 1 min jogging & 1 min brisk walking	20 Alternate 2 mins jogging & 2 mins brisk walking	25 Alternate 5 mins jogging & 5 mins brisk walking
20 Alternate 1 min jogging & 1 min brisk walking	5 mins brisk walking 10 mins jogging 5 mins brisk walking	5 mins brisk walking 15 mins jogging 5 mins brisk walking	20 mins jogging

WARMING UP AND STRETCHING EXERCISES

Here are 6 simple stretching exercises. Do them at least 3 times a week and you'll begin to feel your body becoming more supple and relaxed. You should also do them to warm up before starting on anything more vigorous.

Do all stretching exercises slowly and smoothly. Repeat each one 8 to 12 times. Doing them more times or more quickly *won't* have any extra benefit. *You don't need to do 12 on the first day.* Just do as many as you are comfortable doing and gradually build up.

If you have trouble with back pain it might be advisable to see your doctor first. In any case do these exercises very gently.

1 Arm circling
This is to maintain suppleness in your shoulders.

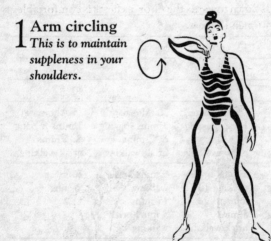

✳ Stand tall and relaxed with your arms at your sides. Slowly circle your right shoulder backwards. Repeat with your left shoulder and continue on alternate sides.

* Place your right hand on your right shoulder. Move your elbow forwards, up, and back, in a circle. Repeat with your left elbow, and continue on alternate sides.

* Start with your arms straight at your sides. Keep your hips facing forwards and move your right arm forward, up, and back, to form a large circle. Repeat with the left arm and continue on alternate sides.

* Any of these arm circles can be done with both arms together.

2 Forward bending
This is to stretch the muscles in your shoulders, trunk and legs.

* Stand tall and relaxed. Stretching through your whole body, reach up towards the ceiling with your fingertips. Then, letting yourself bend at the hips and the knees, slowly bring your hands down towards the floor, as far as is comfortable. Straighten up and repeat.

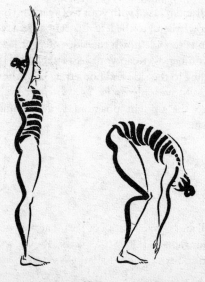

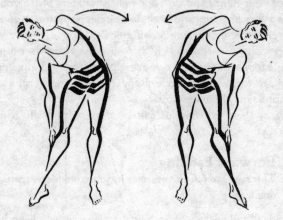

3 Side bending

This is to stretch the muscles in your sides and help keep your spine flexible.

✱ Stand tall and relaxed with your feet apart and hands at your sides. Slowly bend to the left and right alternately, allowing your hands to slide down the sides of your legs. Stand tall in between bends. Keep your legs straight. Make sure you are bending to the side and not letting your shoulders drop forwards. Move only as far as you can comfortably and return to the upright position. Don't bounce into the movement.

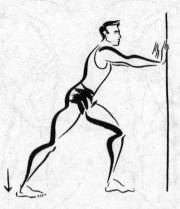

4 Calf stretching
This is to stretch your calves and keep your ankles mobile.

* Stand facing a wall, at arm's length from it. Place your hands on the wall for support and stretch your right leg out straight behind you with the ball of your foot on the floor, and your toes pointing towards the wall. Gently push your right heel towards the floor allowing your left leg to bend as necessary (but no further than is shown in the picture).

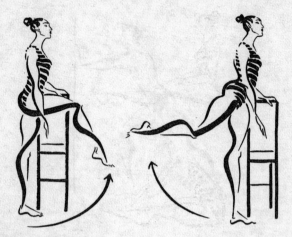

5 Leg swinging
This is to keep your hips mobile and to stretch the thigh muscles.

✱ Stand tall and relaxed with your weight on your left leg. Rest your left hand on the back of a chair for support, if necessary. Now swing your right leg forwards and backwards in a relaxed pendulum action. Gradually take your leg as high as you comfortably can, keeping your body fairly upright and letting your right knee bend. Repeat with your left leg.

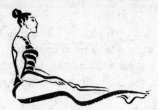

6 Ankle reaching
This is to stretch your lower back and the backs of your thighs.

* Sit on the floor with your legs straight in front of you and your knees as near to the floor as is comfortable. Place your hands on top of your thighs. Slowly and smoothly slide your hands down your legs as far as you can comfortably reach. Return to the upright position and repeat. Do not bounce into the movement.

SHAPING YOUR BODY

Try to do these strength and toning exercises every day, or at least twice a week. Don't push yourself too hard to start with. Five or 6 repeats will probably be plenty to start with. Build up gently and gradually to about 20 repeats.

1 Breast firming
These exercises strengthen mostly upper arms, shoulders and chest. They will help to firm up your bust.

✱ Stand at arm's length from a wall. Place your hands shoulder width apart on the wall. Now bend your arms until your forehead touches the wall. Then push yourself away again until your arms are straight.

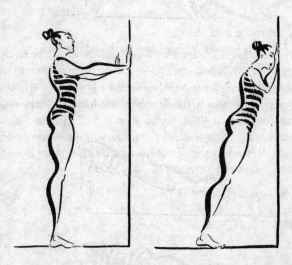

* Kneel on all fours. Move your hands forward slightly and take most of your weight onto them. Bend your arms and lower the top half of your body towards the floor. Only go as far as is comfortable, and be careful not to sag in the middle. Straighten your arms again and return to the starting position.

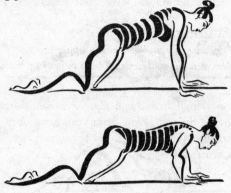

* If you can do the kneeling press-ups easily you may be ready to attempt a full press-up. Follow the instructions above but alter the starting position by lifting your knees off the floor, so that your weight is supported on your hands and toes and your body is in a straight line.

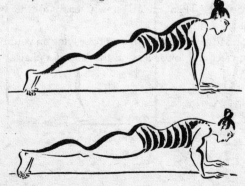

2 Tummy trimming
Weak muscles in the stomach and back put extra strain on your spine. These exercises will help to strengthen your stomach muscles, flatten any bulges and improve your posture.

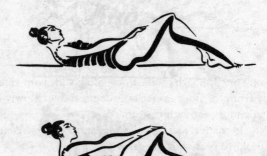

* Lie on your back with your knees bent. Put your hands on the top of your thighs. Lifting just your head and shoulders off the floor, slide your fingers along your thighs as far as is comfortable. Then uncurl slowly back to the lying position.
* As an alternative you can do this exercise lying on your back with your feet and lower legs on the seat of a chair.

3 Hips and thighs
Leg-lifts strengthen and firm your hips and back.

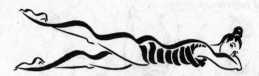

* Lie on your stomach on the floor. Slowly lift your right leg away from the floor, as far as is comfortable. Slowly let it down and repeat with the other leg.
* As an alternative, start on all fours and slowly stretch one leg back. Repeat with the other leg.

> *The following leg exercises will help you tone up and strengthen your thighs, calves and bottom. They are particularly important for older people.*

* Sit on a firm kitchen chair. Stand up without using your hands and without leaning forward too much, if you can. Make sure your legs straighten completely. Sit down again and repeat. Gradually progress just to touching the chair instead of sitting down each time.
* Stand at the bottom of a flight of stairs. Step up onto the first step, making sure you straighten both legs. Step down again. Do this with alternate legs.

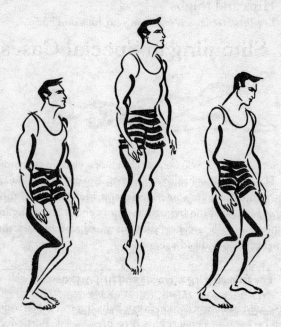

* Stand with your feet together and your knees slightly bent. Spring up, landing with your feet comfortably apart and your knees bent. Now spring up again, landing with your feet together. Repeat as a continuous movement – apart, together, apart, together. Once you can do about 20 repeats, this exercise will also help to build up your stamina.

22 Slimming in Special Cases

In general, whoever you are, you can lose weight in the same way: *The BBC Diet* is healthy for everyone. But at particular stages of life there are some special considerations and this chapter highlights the important points about slimming in childhood and adolescence; pregnancy and after childbirth; the menopause and old age.

SLIMMING AND CHILDREN

You should be concerned that your baby doesn't get fat; one of the best ways to ensure this is to breast-feed. Bottle-fed babies are more likely to get overweight than breast-fed ones. If your baby is fat, discuss what you can do with your health visitor. Your view of what a fat baby is needs to be confirmed by a professional. Never think of putting a baby or toddler on a diet before talking things over with your doctor or health visitor.

Remember that there's an increased risk that overweight children will become overweight adults (see p. 37). So we should take overweight children seriously; it's not justified simply to assume that fat children will 'grow out of it'. Certainly it seems that the majority will; but a sizeable number will become fat adults too.

It seems that often, the very obese people who need to be treated for their overweight at hospital clinics begin to become overweight when they are children. Remember that if you or your spouse are overweight (and particularly if you both are) then your children are more likely to become overweight. It's not inevitable, but you should try to do something about it before it happens.

It's very useful to get your child to fill in a food diary (see pp. 72–3) – you could make it fun and treat it as a game. Pay particular attention to what's eaten at school meals and at break-times. Then what you need to be doing is changing the diet of the whole family to a more healthy and less fattening one. This will have benefits for you as well, but it will have particular benefits for your children. If your child is overweight, you need to think in the same way as you would for yourself: how can I reduce fat and sugar in his or her diet and how can I increase the fibre? It's unfair to expect a child to change his or her eating habits when the rest of the family doesn't – this is an ideal opportunity for the whole family to switch to a healthier diet. The principles outlined in *The BBC Diet* apply to children as much as adults but the one thing that should be mentioned is that children under two derive many of their calories from milk; it's wise to give them whole milk until this age and then get them used to semi-skimmed. Start giving them skimmed milk only after the age of five.

The problem of overweight in children is more complicated than in adults because weight gain does depend partly on height gain. It is important to determine whether the child's pattern of eating or exercise is unusual. It's advisable therefore to take your doctor's advice if you are worried about your child's weight.

SLIMMING AND ADOLESCENTS

Attempts to slim obese young teenagers have sometimes been discouraged because it was thought that the development of anorexia nervosa would be encouraged, particularly in girls. But anorexia is not caused by slimming and there is certainly no reason not to encourage teenagers – overweight or not – to follow a healthy and therefore non-fattening eating pattern.

Anorexia nervosa occurs in about 1 per cent of girls aged 16–18 years and is very uncommon, though not unknown, in boys. It's really caused by a distortion of body image, coupled with, it's thought, a rejection of the process of sexual maturity. Those who suffer from anorexia may be of normal weight or even thin, but think that they are fat and need to lose weight.

Anorexia nervosa and the related disease bulimia need specialist medical treatment. But fear of these diseases is not a reason for a teenager who is actually overweight not to try to lose weight.

SLIMMING IN PREGNANCY AND AFTER CHILDBIRTH

The average weight gain in pregnancy is about 27 lb (12.5 kg). About 15 lb (7 kg) of this is water; 2 lb (1 kg) is protein of which half is in the baby; and about 10 lb (4 kg) of fat is added to the mother's energy stores as a reserve to support the supply of milk during breast-feeding. In pregnancy, especially, the quality of the food, and not its quantity, is important. There appears to be a small increase in food intake in early pregnancy and little change thereafter. There's a fall in physical activity in late pregnancy. In addition, it seems an alteration in metabolic efficiency occurs, which enables the extra fat to be laid down despite the increasing needs of the baby.

The total energy cost of pregnancy and breast-feeding has been calculated at 80 800 calories! It's certainly been shown that the baby is not at a disadvantage, and indeed may be at an advantage, if the mother gains less weight than 27 lbs (12.5 kg). Indeed, most doctors believe that a weight gain of about 15 lb (7 kg) overall would be most beneficial for the baby and, in this case, the mother's weight after delivery would be less than before pregnancy. Against this must be set the other known fact that there's a possibility of the growth of the baby being affected if the mother is malnourished.

This is quite unlikely in this country if the mother begins her pregnancy healthy and well-nourished. In fact, compared with the young of other species, the human baby is quite small and slow-growing and so isn't a great nutritional burden to the mother.

So what conclusion can one come to? Obviously, you're going to be attending ante-natal clinics and taking your doctor's advice. If you are overweight, pregnancy may be an opportunity to control your weight. Talk to your doctor about it. Certainly you can follow the guidelines of *The BBC Diet*, but don't restrict the quantity of the food you eat. (You'll probably find it difficult to restrict anyway, as during pregnancy the appetite increases.) If you're eating the quantity you wish, but cutting down fatty and sugary food and increasing food rich in fibre, you should end up after delivery weighing less than before you became pregnant.

There is a tendency for women to become fatter with increasing age, but the number of children you have, on the whole, makes only a negligible contribution to this weight increase. This is true for most women, though there are some, who are already the most overweight, for whom pregnancy is associated with a much greater weight gain.

When you're breast-feeding, the energy required to produce the milk each day comes to about 675 calories. This energy is normally supplied by breaking down the extra 10 lb (4 kg) or so of fat which has been laid down during pregnancy. This is another good reason for breast-feeding – you're helping yourself and your baby not to get fat.

Even if food has been restricted during pregnancy, this doesn't seem to affect lactation. Again, following the guidelines of *The BBC Diet* is perfectly safe when you're breast-feeding. Certainly 'eating for two' is no excuse to eat excessively – one of the two is very tiny!

SLIMMING AND THE MENOPAUSE

Sex hormones do certainly influence the amount of fat in the body, as evidenced by the differences in body fat between men and women. Women who have had their ovaries removed (usually as part of a hysterectomy) frequently tend to put on weight.

In the United Kingdom, women as a group tend to put on weight around the time of the menopause, but whether this is because of metabolic, physiological or social reasons is unclear.

Whatever the reason, you need to be particularly careful about watching your weight around the time of the menopause. You can safely and healthily follow all the recommendations of *The BBC Diet*.

SLIMMING AND OLDER PEOPLE

We seem to have accepted in Britain that it's normal to put on weight as we get older. It's certainly common but it isn't normal. There's no need to put on extra weight as we get older and there's every reason to make sure we don't – we'll feel better and be more mobile for one thing. How you look becomes less important as you get older and even how long you live becomes less important – what becomes increasingly important is the quality of life you have. If you're fat, your quality of life will certainly be improved if you lose weight.

You can follow *The BBC Diet* no matter how old you are. And remember you can – and should – take some exercise no matter what your age is. Look at chapter 21 to see all the benefits exercise brings no matter what your age.

23 Great Expectations

How much weight will you lose and how quickly? In chapter 1 you've read the stories of just a very few of the people who've lost weight on *The BBC Diet*. Some of them have had quite spectacular weight loss.

There's no reason why you can't join them, but how much weight you lose and how quickly depends on many factors.

* Weight loss is always more rapid at the beginning of a diet but remember there is a difference between losing weight and losing fat (see pp. 45–6). When your weight loss slows down from then on you are losing proportionately more fat.

* On the whole, men will find it easier to lose weight than women. (Sorry about that, but I didn't invent the rules of the game!)

* People who are very overweight will find it easier to lose weight than those who just have to shift a few pounds.

* Your weight loss will, of course, be faster if you start doing some exercise in addition to cutting the calories (see chapter 21).

These factors are the same with any diet and there's no getting round them. To sustain and continue your weight loss, you need to change some of those habits which got you fat in the first place, then you will slim steadily but surely until you're down to your ideal.

On any diet which effectively cuts calories, the pattern of weight loss is the same. The only difference is that there are easy and harder ways to cut calories – and *The BBC Diet* is a very easy way.

Here's what the pattern of weight loss looks like (any variations are due to the way an individual's body reacts and to the points made on pp. 39–41):

The first 2 or 3 weeks	Rapid weight loss of between 7–12 lb (3–5.5 kg)
The next 2 weeks	Weight loss of 2–4 lb (1–1.75 kg) a week
The next month	Weight loss of 1–2 lb (450 g–1 kg) a week

From then on, the weight loss should be a steady 1–2 lb (450g-1 kg) a week until you reach your ideal weight.

Remember that even on a total starvation diet – which is of course dangerous – the weight loss, after the initial rapid phase, would only be 4 lb (1.75 kg) a week (see p. 51). The good news is, even if you continued to lose weight at 'only' 1 lb (450 g) a week, in 3 months you would have lost a further stone (6.35 kg).

And you can do it – look back at some of the success stories in chapter 1.

THE PLATEAU

Some people find that they begin to diet, all goes well for a couple of weeks, they're really pleased with their weight loss and then – arrrgh! A week or two goes by with no weight loss at all. Yet they're still sticking to the diet and they can't understand it.

This is the so-called 'plateau' or levelling-off effect and it certainly can happen. Don't be discouraged. All it means is that your body's metabolism is adjusting to your being on a diet. Don't give up but stick to exactly the same diet and don't be tempted to start crash dieting in an attempt to beat your metabolism: you can't. If you have patience and carry on with your diet, you will go through this 'plateau' and start to lose weight again.

Taking more exercise is a particularly good idea at this time as it should make any 'plateau' phase shorter. But don't worry about it: many people who have made really spectacular weight losses have gone through one or two 'plateaux' before they've got there. Remember how many years it may have taken you to put on this weight. What's a month or two in taking it off?

24 Now You've Got It Off, Keep It Off!

At last, you've reached your goal – the new, slim you. Think of your achievement as an investment – you don't want to throw it away by starting to get fat again.

If you've followed *The BBC Diet*, you'll now have a great practical knowledge of why we put on weight and how we can lose it. Applying that knowledge is your insurance policy against getting fat again.

You need to keep in your mind the following maintenance guidelines. They are similar to but less strict than the losing weight guidelines in chapter 9 which you used if you followed The DIY BBC Diet. They again cover the three areas: fat, sugar and fibre. Try to get familiar with these guidelines.

WHERE'S THE FAT?

Let's remind ourselves again where the fat comes from in the average British diet:

25 per cent from meat and meat products
21 per cent from butter and margarine
14 per cent from cooking oils and fats
11 per cent from milk
7 per cent from biscuits, cakes and pastries
7 per cent from cream and cheese
15 per cent from other foods

We'll consider how we cut down – or cut out – the fat in each of these categories. Remember that cutting down fat is the single most important thing we can do in our continued fight against the flab. Weight-for-weight, fat contains twice as many calories as protein and carbohydrate.

Cutting down fat from meat and meat products

* Cut out meat products like pies, sausages and pâtés completely, if you can. The only 'safe' meat is lean pieces that you can identify. If you don't want to cut out these products completely, look for the lower-fat versions of them.

* Cut off any visible fat on meat. Choose lean cuts, e.g. leg of lamb rather than shoulder. Your portion size of lean meat should be about 3–4 oz (75–100 g).

* White chicken meat is very lean provided you remove the skin; this gets rid of most of the fat and half the calories. Your portion size should be 4–6 oz (100–175 g). Turkey and game are also low in fat; on the other hand, duck and goose are quite fatty.

* Eat more fish. White fish is extremely low in fat. Portion size here can be about 5–7 oz (150–200 g). Fish like herrings and mackerel contain more fat but when grilled are not too high in calories. Continue to choose tinned fish like sardines and tuna packed in brine or water rather than oil – this almost halves the calories.

* Always grill rather than fry meat – this very significantly reduces the calories. Alternatively, microwave or poach in water or skimmed milk, or steam.

* If using mince, choose the leanest you can buy. Pour off all the fat after 'dry frying' (see p. 86), or cover with water, bring slowly to the boil, simmer gently for a

couple of minutes, pour off the now fatty water and then proceed with your recipe.

* In casseroles and other similar dishes you are making for yourself, cut down the amount of meat you would normally use. Remember even lean red meat has a significant fat content. To supplement the meat, add pulses like beans, lentils, split peas or chick peas.

Cutting down the fat from butter and margarine

* This fat is rather easier to identify and therefore to avoid. Remember, on average, almost one quarter of the fat in our diet comes from these sources.

* Cut out butter and margarine as completely as you can. If you want to continue with butter or margarine, spread it thinly and use it sparingly.

* Substitute a low-fat spread such as Gold or Outline. Continue to make sandwiches with the low-fat spread on one of the slices of bread rather than on both and not using any if the filling is moist.

Cutting down the fat from cooking oils and fats

* You'll be cutting these down to the very minimum by grilling rather than frying.

* When you do want to fry, you can 'dry fry' (see p. 86) using no oil at all. Alternatively, you could use a very small amount of oil. You should be able to fry an onion in 1–2 teaspoonfuls of oil. This could, of course, be a dish for 2–4 people so the amount of oil per person will be very tiny.

* Remember, 1 tablespoonful of oil contains 120 calories.

This is why you should measure out your oil in teaspoonfuls (40 calories) and certainly don't pour it from the bottle – one generous slurp could be a quarter of your calorie target for the day!

* For your health's sake and that of your family, use polyunsaturated oil rather than hard cooking fats or oils just labelled 'cooking oil'. Find a 'named oil' like sunflower, safflower or groundnut as these, particularly the first two, are high in polyunsaturates. Olive oil, which is also healthy (high in monounsaturates) is strongly flavoured and can therefore make its mark in a dish in very small quantities.

* Remember mayonnaise is largely oil and so packed with calories. Use instead the variety of yoghurt dressings on pp. 325–6). If you want to have mayonnaise very occasionally mix it half and half with low-fat natural yoghurt. This is still rich and satisfying but has half the calories.

* When you're making chips for the family (and very, very occasionally for yourself) you can cut down the fat considerably. Cut your chips thickly (so that weight-for-weight there's a lower surface area to absorb the fat) and then fry them quickly in hot oil. (Hot oil seeps into the chips less than cooler oil.) Again, use an oil high in polyunsaturates and don't keep re-using it (which causes it to become saturated fat). Finally, shake off as much oil as possible and then, before serving, drain the chips on kitchen paper to get rid of any remaining fat. As an alternative, oven chips can contain up to 40 per cent fewer calories than home-made chips. Look for the ones which are cooked in sunflower oil.

Cutting down the fat from milk

* This is easy: use only skimmed milk.

* Semi-skimmed milk has virtually no fat at all. When you've reached your ideal weight, you may be very happy staying with skimmed milk and that would be excellent. If you do want something a little richer, you could go to semi-skimmed milk. Don't go back to whole milk.

Cutting down the fat from biscuits, cakes and pastries

* The ideal is to stop eating these altogether and just have them as a very occasional treat.

* The other advantage of cutting this fat source is that it's all here as sweet fat. You cut the fat and the sugar at the same time.

* Fresh fruit is the healthy and slimming alternative to these products.

Cutting down the fat from cream and cheese

* You know what to do about cream: it's a 'no-no' food while you want to lose weight and very much a 'sometimes' food once you've reached your ideal weight.

* Remember the tasty, healthy and low-fat substitutes for cream — low-fat natural yoghurt, Greek yoghurt and fromage frais (see p. 90).

* Remember that Cheddar-type cheeses are one-third fat. Stilton and cream cheeses are nearly half fat. Avoid these as much as you can.

* Softer cheeses like Brie, Camembert and Edam are about a quarter fat.

* The lower-fat Cheddar-type cheese on sale usually contains less than half the fat of conventional Cheddar – about 14 per cent fat. There are also now many low-fat versions of soft cheeses. However, it's best to use these products as a way of further cutting down your calories rather than as a way of eating more cheese!

* Cottage cheese – cultivate a taste for it and eat it as much as you like!

* When cooking with cheese, use a stronger flavoured variety, perhaps adding a little mustard and that way you will need less cheese.

Cutting down the rest of the fat in our diet

There is a wide variety of other fat sources in our diet but we only need to think about the most significant.

* Nuts and salted snacks, crisps and all those other savoury snacks are high in fat. You need to cut them out completely or keep them for very occasional treats.

* Although there are only about 80 calories in a medium-sized egg, 3–4 eggs a week is a good balance to aim for.

WHERE'S THE SUGAR?

Remembering the staggering daily calories we each obtain from sugar, it is well worth keeping your sugar consumption under a tight rein (see pp. 66–7).

* Continue not to take sugar in tea or coffee. You really can wean yourself off it. As for artificial sweeteners, remember that Sorbitol, used in most diabetic sweets and chocolates, contains as many calories as sugar. Make sure you're using a slimmer's sweetener.

* Continue to cut out fizzy canned drinks. Even though you can get low-cal drinks it is better to drink sparkling mineral water with ice and lemon, or unsweetened fruit juices.

* Continue to cut out sweet snacks, biscuits, chocolates, cakes or keep them for very occasional treats – eat fresh fruit instead.

* Continue to use tinned fruit packed in natural fruit juice rather than packed in sugar syrup.

* Don't go back to adding sugar to your breakfast cereal – keep checking labels in case it's been added already.

* Continue to read labels before you consume anything from a packet or tin. You need to keep being aware of just what you're getting. Pick those 'reduced-sugar' and 'no added sugar' products every time but still go sparingly with sweet products even if the label proclaims 'less sugar'.

* Keep up the good work in gradually cutting down the sugar you add to cakes, pies etc. when you're baking things at home. Remember, you're only meant to partake occasionally in these treats and by cutting down the amount of sugar in your family's diet in this way you're also doing them a favour.

WHERE'S THE FIBRE?

Remind yourself of the best sources of fibre by looking at the list on p. 105. Keep these in mind when planning your meals and try and put the following into practice.

* Try to start the day with muesli or a wholemeal breakfast cereal with no added sugar.

* Try to eat at least 4 slices of wholemeal bread a day now

you're at your ideal weight. Remember that wholemeal is richer in fibre than just 'brown' or 'wheatmeal' bread.

* Make sure your main meal is still accompanied by a fibre-rich helping of one of the following:

  potatoes (up to 8 oz, 225 g), scrubbed not peeled, either baked or boiled

  brown rice (up to 3 oz, 75 g)

  wholewheat pasta (up to 3 oz, 75 g)

  bulgar wheat (up to 3 oz, 75 g)

* Continue to try to eat a portion of peas or beans or other pulses once a day.

* Eat at least one other portion of fresh vegetables a day. All vegetables contain some fibre, but the really fibre-rich ones are green leafy vegetables like spinach.

* Eat two or three pieces of fresh fruit every day. Remember not to eat too much dried fruit unless it's been soaked and cooked.

WHERE ELSE CAN WE CUT CALORIES?

Remember, alcohol. The average person will be taking perhaps 10 per cent of their daily calorie consumption from alcohol. This is drinking perhaps two or three drinks a day. You need to be careful how much alcohol you continue to drink both for the sake of your weight, and your health (see p. 107).

ADAPTING RECIPES

If you keep 'thinking fat and thinking sugar' you should be able to cut the calorie count of many of your favourite recipes.

* Try cutting the fat and the sugar in your baking recipes.

* Whenever there's fat in any other recipe always halve it, at *least*. Better still, try it without.

* Substitute skimmed milk for whole milk and fromage frais or low-fat natural yoghurt for cream (see p. 90).

* In all chicken recipes remove the skin.

* With soups, stocks and casseroles always try to prepare in advance. If you leave them to cool, the fat rises to the top and can then be spooned off.

* After frying, pour off any fat and perhaps also blot it up with kitchen paper.

* But, preferably, of course you won't be frying! If you don't grill then 'dry fry' (see p. 86). Or, if you must, stir-fry in minimal oil and blot up the excess later.

SOME FINAL THOUGHTS

Monitor your weight carefully. Weigh yourself once a week. Remember that fat creeps up slowly, pound by pernicious pound. If we only put on 4 oz (100 g) a week – that's nearly a stone (6.35 kg) in a year.

By following *The BBC Diet*, you will have become used to low-fat, low-sugar, high-fibre food; you'll have discovered that it's enjoyable. Hopefully, some of the new food habits you've developed will have become ingrained and will last a lifetime. Remember that although *The BBC Diet* is the very best diet for losing weight, it's also the very best for becoming healthy and keeping healthy. Try to incorporate as many of its guidelines into your life 'post-diet' – and remember, getting your family and particularly your children into healthy eating ways is one of the biggest gifts you can give them.

What if you can't face life without chocolate, cream

cakes, fish and chips? Don't despair. Remember that no food can make you fat if you only eat it once a week. What you eat most of the time is what makes you fat, not what you eat occasionally. Eat sensibly, trying to follow the guidelines for six (or better six and a half) days a week and then eat what you fancy for one or two meals a week. Of course, you could find that healthy and slimming food becomes your favourite food – it does happen!

For Your
Personal Records

FOOD DIARY

When?	Where?	What?	With whom?

What were you doing?	Were you hungry?	How did you feel?	Comment

```
                    I,
           promise myself that I shall lose
        After I have lost the first     I shall buy
                    myself a
        After I have lost the next   I shall buy myself
                        a
           And after I have lost the whole    I shall buy
                    myself a
```

```
        I,          promise to lose    stone
            and I,        promise to help
           After she has lost   , I shall give her
                        a
    After     has lost the next   , I shall give
                    and after    has lost
            the whole        I shall give
```

Date	Weight

Date	Weight

Date	Bust/chest	Waist	Hips	Thighs	Upper arm

Date	Bust/chest	Waist	Hips	Thighs	Upper arm

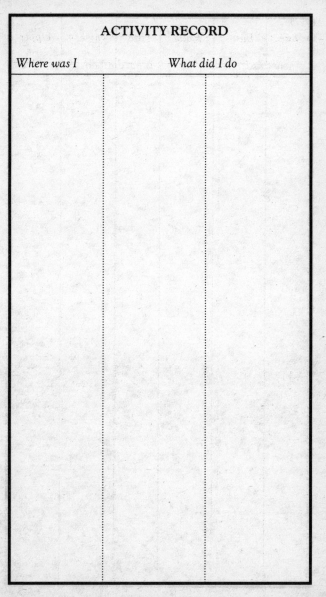

ACTIVITY RECORD

Where was I	What did I do

ACTIVITY RECORD

Where was I	What did I do

EXERCISE DIARY

Time	Exercise	How Long

EXERCISE DIARY

Time	Exercise	How Long

Index of Recipes